Expert Report Writing
in Toxicology

Expert Report Writing in Toxicology

Forensic, Scientific and Legal Aspects

Michael D. Coleman
Aston University, Birmingham, UK

WILEY Blackwell

This edition first published 2014 © 2014 by John Wiley & Sons, Ltd

Registered Office
John Wiley & Sons, Ltd, The Atrium, Southern Gate, Chichester, West Sussex, PO19 8SQ, UK

Editorial Offices
9600 Garsington Road, Oxford, OX4 2DQ, UK
The Atrium, Southern Gate, Chichester, West Sussex, PO19 8SQ, UK
111 River Street, Hoboken, NJ 07030-5774, USA

For details of our global editorial offices, for customer services and for information about how to apply for permission to reuse the copyright material in this book please see our website at www.wiley.com/wiley-blackwell.

Library of Congress Cataloging-in-Publication Data

Coleman, Michael D., author.
 Expert report writing in toxicology: forensic, scientific, and legal aspects / Michael D. Coleman.
   p. ; cm.
 Includes index.
 ISBN 978-1-118-43237-2 (cloth) – ISBN 978-1-118-43214-3 (pbk.)
 I. Title.
 [DNLM: 1. Forensic Toxicology. 2. Expert Testimony. 3. Manufactured Materials–toxicity.
4. Occupational Exposure–adverse effects. 5. Pesticides–toxicity. 6. Writing. W 750]
 RA1228
 614′.13–dc23
                                        2013046819

A catalogue record for this book is available from the British Library.

Wiley also publishes its books in a variety of electronic formats. Some content that appears in print may not be available in electronic books.

Set in 10.5/12.5pt Times by SPi Publisher Services, Pondicherry, India
Printed and bound in Singapore by Markono Print Media Pte Ltd

1 2014

This book is dedicated to Walter Drozd and Brian Odell

Contents

Contents

Preface

Most of us at one time or another have complained about issues relating to our workplace. It might be too hot or too cold; perhaps the chairs are uncomfortable and our colleagues and line managers are too annoying, aggressive, passive or uncaring. Perhaps the majority of us feel undervalued and under-rewarded for our efforts. However, one issue that relatively few of us in the developed world are likely to be worried about currently is whether our occupation might lead us to an early and unpleasant death due to a disease or condition brought about by our work and its environment. This is partly because of the vast changes in work patterns which have occurred over the past half-century in developed countries. Many of our great-grandparents and grandparents toiled in hard physical work, which might have meant jobs in areas such as heavy industry, manufacturing, farming, fishing, mining or construction. Many of these occupations caused severe and long-term impact on health, and in many cases the individuals concerned did not even live to retirement age. We still need the products of industry such as steel and aluminium for our cars, and we use myriad manufactured goods, eat fresh produce and fish, burn coal, move into new houses and use new roads. However, as a society, we have effectively 'outsourced' many of these difficult and hazardous occupations to other, usually developing countries.

Regarding those physical occupations in hazardous environments that remain in the developed world, the suffering of previous generations has led to the creation of an effective, complex, yet sometimes ridiculed Health and Safety apparatus which has greatly diminished, but sadly not eliminated, the risks of ill-health arising from occupation. Chapter 1 of this book outlines some of the historical milestones in the evolution of our occupational health knowledge, awareness and practice. This chapter also charts the rise and fall of various industries, as they created wealth, but also human misery, in terms of their widespread toxic impact on workers' health and life expectancy. This introductory chapter also outlines the notion that whilst hard-won experience led to detailed frameworks of Health and Safety practice that are now usually adhered to in the developed world, this is far from the case in the emerging manufacturing powerhouses of the Far East.

Despite our progress in Occupational Health in the developed world, there remains a substantial number of individuals whose health has been irreparably damaged by their occupation. The second chapter begins with the main features of the process whereby some recognition can be obtained for their suffering, as well as financial redress for loss of earnings and any necessary support for attainment of some quality of life. Whilst recognition and compensation can arise from some mutual agreement between former employee and employer, court action, or the threat of it, might be necessary for a final settlement. Naturally, much documentation is necessary for such actions to proceed, but expert reports are amongst the most important material needed to propel a case. From the perspective of the claimant, it is as if they wish to communicate to the court initially, *look at me now and my medical impairments*, which are dealt with by the medical report or reports. Subsequently, the claimant wants to establish *how this happened to me*, which is covered by other expert reports, notably on causation. Clearly a medical examination will provide a picture of the claimant's health impairments, which is usually relatively straightforward to describe and justify. Causation, in terms of how a substance or substances led the claimant to his or her current plight, may be much harder to establish, and the main purpose of this book is to provide the aspiring expert report writer with my own experience to illuminate this area.

It is not always easy for solicitors mounting cases to recruit relevant experts to contribute reports on causation. If causation cannot be established, then clearly the court will not be convinced and cases may not proceed because of a shortage of appropriate expertise. This may be particularly important in cases where the claimant is suffering from life-threatening health issues and may not have the luxury of time to pursue a case. Experts might be difficult to recruit due to a general shortage of qualified individuals in a particularly narrow field, or perhaps due to sheer pressure of other commitments. Indeed, an expert's credibility in part stems from validation supplied by their continued employment by their institution so their commitment to their employer's demands is, of course, paramount. It is also possible that prospective experts with the appropriate research interests and experience, as well as the relevant writing and oral skills, may hesitate to offer their services for different reasons. These might include a lack of familiarity with the legal context and framework of report drafting, or insufficient confidence in whether they already possess appropriate skills and knowledge to draft an effective report. Chapter 2 supplies some guidance as to how the expert report fits into the current legal process and how their work is evaluated and employed by the claimant's legal team, as well as the court.

The remaining chapters provide case histories where I have written reports as part of cases in various broadly themed areas, ranging from exposure to solvents and adhesives (Chapter 3), petrochemical-induced cases of bladder cancer (Chapter 4), as well as the impact of herbicides and insecticides (Chapter 5). In contrast, rather than focus on the occupational issues of the manufacturers of imported goods, Chapter 6 features the toxicity of some of the products of Far Eastern economic success. Whilst this book is not intended to be a toxicology text, I have striven to make the toxicological issues as accessible as possible to enable the arguments to be weighed and criticised. In addition, it is hoped that the book may be useful to all interested participants of the process of establishing causation in occupational toxicity proceedings.

The case histories are taken from some of the reports I prepared and submitted from 1997 to 2009. Indeed, depending on the reader's own expertise and experience, they will form their own opinion of the quality of the reports I compiled, and they may well feel that they could have constructed considerably better drafted and more convincing arguments, given the same starting information. If this is the case, then this book will have achieved one of its aims, which is to encourage those who could 'assist the court' to do so and to do a better job than I could do. Of course, in any given case, neither the medical experts nor the court or the causation report writing can restore the health of the individual concerned. However, contributing one's expertise towards achieving justice for a claimant is not only worthwhile, in terms of bringing recognition for their plight and others in the same position, but it also contributes to the evolution of the developed world's knowledge of Health and Safety. In addition, the publicity which sometimes surrounds cases also highlights the impact of old and hazardous industries, but also the effects of new processes on health which were not anticipated or expected.

My only personal experience of the damage occupation can do to health was the impact on my father of his service as a Wireless Telegraphist in the Royal Navy in World War II. Aside from surviving four years of Arctic weather, he had many lucky escapes, such as watching a torpedo from a U-Boat pass under his ship, a bout of persistent friendly fire by a US Air Force Lightning fighter, as well as a perilously close small arms attack whilst at anchor in Norway after the Germans had officially withdrawn. Ironically, it was his day-to-day work of high-frequency radio signalling, as well as using rifle fire to 'pot' mines during sweeping processes, that caused lifelong and severe impairment to his hearing, which deteriorated to virtually nothing towards the end of his life. Whilst he was, of course, grateful to survive, his deafness often made his personal and professional lives profoundly difficult, although he bore it with fortitude.

Chapter 6 considers the developing world's extremely uneven awareness of occupational health damage, albeit indirectly, through the toxicity of their products which have reached the United Kingdom. The Epilogue reflects on the gradual improvement of developing world Health and Safety, through advances in education and prosperity. Having spent the last few decades using manufacturing to generate wealth to attain Western living standards, it is to be hoped that developing countries will also see the necessity of adopting Health and Safety structures and practices, as well as improving existing ones, so that future manufacturing can be as safe for their workforces, as it should be sustainable and profitable. Every effort has been made to make this book as accurate as possible, but nothing and nobody is perfect. I am grateful to my wife Clare, my mother Jean and my family for their support during the preparation of the manuscript, and I hope that the book will be of use.

M.D. Coleman, D.Sc.
September 2013

'If I am given six hours to cut down a tree,
I will spend four hours sharpening the axe'

Abraham Lincoln (1809–1865)

1
A brief history of occupational toxicology

1.1   Occupational toxin exposure in antiquity

There are several activities essential to a civilised society, such as reliable food production as well as some provision for manufacturing and processing goods and foodstuffs. Whilst farming came comparatively late in human evolution, perhaps 8000–10,000 years BC, manufacturing of some recognisable sort appeared even later, when humans started to mine and process various metals. Of course, recovering metal ores from underground exposes the individual to many physical dangers, such as rock falls, floods and toxic gases. However, the significant energy input required for the extraction and processing of pure metals presented new hazards, such as the hot gases and dangers of the molten product. Many ancient cultures soon developed what we might recognise as a production process, where metals were mined, smelted and processed, including copper and tin, which were eventually combined to make bronze, which was more durable than either metal alone.

Whilst the process of smelting is inherently dangerous, neither copper nor tin is especially directly toxic to man. Indeed, the metal that replaced both of them in tool and weapon manufacture, iron, was also not particularly toxic to process in itself. These metals do not tend to accumulate in the body and cause acute or chronic toxicity during normal processing techniques. Lead, however, is very toxic, and the mining and smelting of this malleable and useful metal were probably the first activities where there were significant acute and chronic toxic hazards encountered during its handling. Lead is usually found as its sulphide (galena), which contains silver, so lead production at first was a by-product of silver recovery. Lead usage was fairly widespread before the ascendancy of the Romans, with many ancient peoples such as the Egyptians, using it for a variety of tasks; these included fishing weights, water piping and the basis of a form of early mascara.

Hippocrates (460–379 BC) [1] was the iconic founder of modern medicine, and it has been thought that he was the first to describe occupational lead poisoning; however, this is not actually true [2] as his description was not as precise as some

Expert Report Writing in Toxicology: Forensic, Scientific and Legal Aspects,
First Edition. Michael D. Coleman.
© 2014 John Wiley & Sons, Ltd. Published 2014 by John Wiley & Sons, Ltd.

authors would have it. The first detailed surviving description of lead intoxication appeared (in verse, apparently) around the second century BC, in the physician and poet Nicander of Colophon's *Alexipharmaca*. As the reach of the Roman Empire extended, by the beginning of the first century AD, lead usage increased dramatically. Indeed, the impact on health of any toxic process is directly related to its scale, and the Romans used vast amounts of lead in their grandiose, but impressively durable building projects. For instance, thousands of tonnes of lead were involved in the construction of a siphon unit in the great aqueduct at Lyon [3]. To supply lead on such a scale meant processing which we would even now recognise as 'industrial'. Consequently, it is not surprising that several Roman figures described the appalling environmental impact of lead processing, as well as the toxicity of the actual processes used for purifying the metal. Towards the end of the first century BC, the architect known today as Vitruvius (Marcus Vitruvius Pollio; ~75 BC to ~ AD 15) described the severe impact on local water supplies of metal processing, and he stated his opposition to the use of lead piping because of its toxicity to the lead workers, as he noticed how pale they looked. The philosopher and scientist Pliny the Elder (Gaius Plinius Secundus; AD 23–79), writing around 70 years later, commented that lead produced 'noxious and deadly fumes' when it was heated and processed. Pliny also designed masks that could be worn by workers to protect them from fumes. Interestingly, as with many toxins, although the dangers of lead were well documented, it continued to be used on a large scale for centuries after the deaths of its early critics. As we know, lead was used in piping and paints until well into the twentieth century and remains in many houses today, carrying drinking water all over the United Kingdom. Whilst it remains useful as a roofing material, perhaps most remarkably, lead was employed in its tetraethyl form for more than 80 years as an anti-detonation agent in fuels, such as petrol (gasoline); unfortunately, vast amounts were released into the atmosphere via this route. Since its removal from fuels in most countries before the year 2000, this source of lead pollution has declined dramatically in developed economies. Currently, lead is much less of a toxic threat than before, although human exposure in foodstuffs will probably never entirely be eradicated.

1.2   The Middle Ages and the Renaissance: The beginnings of modern occupational toxicology

Although always a crucial part of metal industries, mining in general broadened in scope up to the Middle Ages and beyond, as many more materials were actively recovered from deeper and deeper pits. The mining of coal for energy began in earnest after the thirteenth century, and by the end of the fifteenth century, metal mining to support the armaments industry was growing rapidly, as cumbersome cannon evolved towards more intricate hand-firearms. All this increased demand for iron, lead and copper, along with other metals. In 1473, the German physician Ulrich Ellenbog (1435–1499) wrote the landmark paper *Von den gifftigen Besen Tempffen un Reuchen* (On the Poisonous Wicked Fumes and Smokes), where he described the various toxic processes found in the gold mining industry, which involved fuming acids, as well as lead and mercury vapours. A more systematic exploration of mining and its hazards was then made by another German physician *Georgius Agricola* (Georg Bauer; 1494–1555), who developed a lifelong fascination with these subjects. He even bought a share of a silver mine and published several books on mining and various minerals, including *De Re Metallica* [4], which took him more than 20 years to write and was only published after his death. Although the book's main focus is its extraordinary detail of the methods of mining and metal processing of the time, he did investigate and document many of the occupational hazards of mining, including the various types of pneumoconiosis, such as silicosis, as well as other mining health dangers. Agricola is regarded now as a particularly able and methodical scientist, whose enthusiasm (Section 1.11) and understanding of the value of the observation of phenomena in making appropriate deductions were far ahead of his time.

A contemporary of Agricola was the much better known *Paracelsus*, and variations of his ubiquitous quote "All substances are poisons; there is none which is not a poison. The right dose differentiates a poison and a remedy" have adorned many a text and student submission over the centuries. Philippus Theophrastus Aureolus Bombastus von Hohenheim was born in Zurich in 1493. His physician father, Wilhelm Bombast von Hohenheim, became an expert in occupational medicine in much the same way as Agricola, through researching his mining patients' experience. Strongly influenced by his father, young Philippus nevertheless began his studies with the controversial subject of alchemy. Today, the idea of making gold and silver from base metals in an ordinary laboratory sounds as quaint as it is impossible, without the aid of a Nuclear Research Facility. However, as late as the seventeenth century, it was taken deadly seriously, and most of the front rank of scientists at that time, such as Isaac Newton and Robert Boyle, considered themselves alchemists, although in secret.

Philippus Von Hohenheim travelled widely and studied surgery and, through his alchemy activities, chemistry. He began to pioneer the role of chemistry in medicine, rejecting various contemporary 'cures', in favour of a more systematic approach to the use of remedies such as opium, as well as metals such as lead and antimony. He advocated the use of small doses of mercury for syphilis, which was essentially the right idea with the wrong agent, as mercury was eventually proven ineffective for syphilis in the 1940s.

Philippus's ideas were revolutionary for his time, and he is credited with not only 'inventing' pharmacology, through his concept of dose and how its related to response, but also toxicology and even the idea of the 'target organ' for toxicity [5]. Sadly, he managed to combine aggression, certainty, excessive fondness for alcohol, flamboyance and arrogance in his personality and even styled himself *Paracelsus*, or greater than Aulus Cornelius Celsus (~25 BC–AD 50; the Roman author of the medical treatise *De Medicina*). This, combined with contempt for accepted wisdom and a theatrical and sometimes incendiary lecturing style, he ensured that he surpassed all his peers in his ability to make seriously powerful enemies. His drinking led to fatal liver cirrhosis at only 48 years of age, having spent his life challenging and usually failing to defeat medical orthodoxy. However, although he remains controversial to this day, I think it can be said that he made a significant contribution to occupational medicine, not least through his ideas on the specific mechanisms whereby toxins impact the body, as well as a book on miners' diseases. Perhaps it is characteristic of his personality and ambition that he entitled his last major work, *Die Grosse Wundartznei* (*The Great Surgery Book*) of 1536, which restored his fortunes and public image.

As mining became more industrialised, many more debilitating conditions emerged, not least vibration 'white finger' and noise-related deafness, which were linked with cutting and boring machinery, as well as toxicity associated with the fumes of explosives and more recently, underground vehicles. In recent times, whilst mining has all but disappeared in the United Kingdom, it remains a major industry in more than 50 countries worldwide, although fatality rates and occupational disease remain several fold higher than other industries [6, 7]. In the United Kingdom, the legacy of 'black lung', which is the form of pneumoconiosis caused by coal dust, continues to blight and shorten the lives of retired miners. As there remains several hundred years of supply of coal under the United Kingdom, it is likely that this energy will be exploited in the future, not by manual labour, but with the application of new technology applied to underground coal gasification (UCG), which can be carried out from the surface using bore holes. Interestingly, the concept of UCG is far from new; one of its early proponents was Lenin (Vladimir Illych Ulyanov; 1870–1924), who sought in 1913 to make presumably irony-free political capital out of the possible benefits of UCG, in claiming that it would free the proletariat from the dangers of working underground in Tsarist mines [8].

The individual who is regarded now as the father of occupational medicine was the Italian physician and Professor of Medicine at the Universities of Modena and subsequently Padua, Bernadino Ramazzini (1633–1714) [9]. He was the first physician to devote his career to a systematic investigation of over 50 occupations, involving visiting places of work and questioning workers. He exhorted his fellow physicians to routinely enquire after occupation, as well as symptoms. His career culminated in *De Morbis Artificum Diatriba* (*Discourse on the Diseases of Workers*; first edition, 1700, second edition, 1713). This work described many different occupations, their consequences and ideas for alleviation of the damage and the processes that caused it. Importantly, he not only understood that the various noxious materials, gases and vapours to which workers were exposed were actually responsible for their health problems, but also that unusual specific movements and postures required by the occupation contributed to morbidity and mortality. In this latter area, he was the first to recognise repetitive strain injuries, which remain a workplace hazard today. His work anticipated the Industrial Revolution, where manufacturing grew in scale beyond anything that preceded it, involving large numbers of individuals, vast amounts of processing and long periods of exposure to noxious agents, particularly those related to polycyclic aromatic hydrocarbons (PAHs) from coal and petrochemicals.

1.3   The Industrial Revolution

Whilst it is generally accepted that the Industrial Revolution began in Britain, industrialisation and mining expansion occurred in many other countries, and several scientists around Europe made notable contributions to the emerging science of occupational health in the eighteenth century. Gradually, very early concepts, such as Pliny's ideas on protective measures in the workplace, became re-discovered and reinforced, whilst the understanding of specific links between certain toxins and particular conditions and their mechanisms of toxicity, pioneered by Paracelsus, also gathered pace. The brilliant Russian polymath Mikhail Vasilyevich Lomonosov (1711–1765) outlined measures to be taken to ensure occupational safety in mining in a 1763 treatise, although he could be of a similar disposition to Paracelsus and was imprisoned for eight months for abusing his University's administrators (sounds harsh) and was even briefly forcibly retired by the personal order of Catherine The Great. In England, a major step forward in the understanding of how pollutants from a specific occupation can cause permanent and even lethal injury was made by Sir Percivall Pott (1714–1788). Dr Pott was an extremely well-liked, industrious and technically proficient surgeon, who among many other achievements gave his name to a particular type of compound fracture. The image of eighteenth-century medicine is somewhat tarnished by its obsessions with bleeding, purging and, of course, amputation, for a surprisingly wide range of conditions. However, Dr Pott did his very best with what he had, made highly significant additions to medical knowledge and worked tirelessly right up to his death, which was actually hastened by his devotion to his patients.

Today, in the developed world, many developing countries are criticised for allowing dangerous child labour practices; however, from the end of the seventeenth century in England, after being sold to master chimney sweeps by their parents, boys as young as seven years old were sent up naked into extremely cramped chimneys to clean them. They were sometimes 'encouraged' by the sweep lighting a straw fire beneath them [10]. It was not uncommon for these children to die of asphyxiation, and survivors were treated appallingly, with no access to washing facilities. Hence, they would develop scrotal soot warts, which they would sometimes remove by themselves with a knife. These warts would sometimes become cancerous, usually many years later. The idea of employing children in this way was actually considered repugnant even by the end of the eighteenth century, but was not outlawed until 1842 due to the resistance of the master chimney sweeps. Whilst Dr Pott was not the first person to describe the tumours, he made the link between the soot exposure and the tumours, so becoming first to recognise that a malignant disease was caused by a specific occupation [11]. One interesting and important perception he also made was that because the signs of the disease appeared after puberty, it was commonly ascribed by doctors to venereal disease and thus treated with mercury, which of course made things worse. Such understandable misdiagnosis continues today in areas such as idiosyncratic drug reaction, as well as in occupational health, and it still costs the patient time, allowing the disease to progress whilst increasing suffering. As the nineteenth century progressed, it became apparent that scrotal cancers usually presented decades after exposure had finished and although such long lag-times in cancer presentation are still studied even today we do not understand all the processes involved. Interestingly, it was realised as early as the 1890s that chimney sweeps' scrotal cancer was very much an 'English Disease' because in every other country in Europe (even in Scotland), sweeps wore effective protective clothing. Tragically, it took more than a century from the discovery of this cancer towards some means of alleviating it, and right up to the end of the nineteenth century, English sweeps were at an eightfold greater risk of scrotal cancer than other males.

1.4   Petrochemicals: The beginnings

Up to Potts's time, human exposure to PAHs was restricted to environmental coal fire pollution of various sorts, such as in chimney sweeping. As the second half of the nineteenth century progressed, the growing industry of coal distillation produced a variety of different products, ranging from thick, tar-like pitch, to paraffin waxes and various solvent mixes, such as naphtha, creosote and anthracenes. These agents were used as fuels and lubricants of various kinds in many emerging light and heavy industries in England and Europe. It gradually became apparent that workers exposed to these agents, either through their extraction, combustion or usage as lubricants, were suffering from the same scrotal cancers as chimney sweeps. A report by von Volkmann in 1875 [12] revealed that men working with tar distillates were at risk of these cancers. Over the next 25 years or so, many other workers, such as mule spinners in the Lancashire and Yorkshire Cotton Industry, as well as Oil shale workers, were seen to be at risk of petro-chemically induced cancers. The Oil shale business became uneconomic in the 1870s when oil imports began to grow, and only the appearance of modern processing technology and the high price of oil have made shale extraction viable today. The coal tar and oil distillation industry continued to grow from the turn of the century and was particularly well established in Germany, where by 1913 just one factory at Elberfeld run by Bayer employed 8000 workers. It is also worth noting that the number of technically advanced spin-offs of the tar-distillation industry, such as the dye, fuel and tyre industries, was also growing; indeed, the Elberfeld factory employed 330 skilled chemists with university-level educations.

The plight of the mule spinners, however, is a good example of how a combination of specific working practices, environment and toxin exposure can cause an unusual neoplasm. A 'mule' was a long machine invented by Samuel Crompton in the late 1770s that could spin cotton (or other fibres) into yarn, and it was operated by a 'minder' and usually two boy 'piecers' who acted to repair threads when they broke. Each cotton mill might have up to 60 mules, and the basic design did not change until the 1970s when the industry died out in the United Kingdom. From the early 1900s to the 1920s, rates of scrotal cancer in mule spinners reached such levels that strenuous efforts were made to try to understand the process in order to prevent it. By the 1920s, the idea that mineral oils were carcinogenic had reached common medical knowledge, as the carcinogenicity of tar had been clearly demonstrated when it was painted onto rabbits ears [13]. By the 1930s, the carcinogens in tar were narrowed to dibenzanthracenes and 3,4-benzpyrene. In 1926, S.A. Henry (1880–1960) reported that the scrotal cancer developed by the mule spinners was caused by lubricating mineral oil thrown off the machines. Later studies determined that the location of the worker's cancers was probably linked with their tendency during their work to lean across an oily 'faller bar' to repair broken fibres. This was exacerbated by the heat of the mills, where the spinners wore very light clothes which offered no protection against the oil seepage towards the scrotum, and these clothes were extremely contaminated with oil on a daily basis. The skin of the scrotum is 80 times more permeable to toxins than skin on the rest of the body, which promoted the penetration of the oil into tissues. In addition, a mist was formed by the fibres and oil spray, which combined with intense machine noise, suggests a very unpleasant working environment. Indeed, to digress slightly, my closest friend's mother, Mrs Vera Winn, worked in a cotton mill, and she said the only way to communicate was by lip reading; the machines were so loud. The noise levels in many industries were sufficiently high for manufacturers such as Ford in the United Kingdom to make substantial one-off compensation payments to many of their former workers as late as the 1980s.

Returning to the subject of oils, Henry's 1926 report presciently recommended that the oils be replaced by so-called white oils which were pure paraffins and guards should be fitted to the machines to reduce oil splash. Over the next two decades, it took a series of papers by Twort and colleagues in Manchester [14] that not only established that the mineral oils used in mule spinning were carcinogenic, but that if they were used for long periods and subject to heat, such as in use in the mules, even more carcinogenic agents would form through the process known as 'catalytic cracking'. Indeed, this is the basis of petrol and diesel fuel production, where larger polycyclics are broken up into smaller agents. Frequent replacement of the lubricating oil would not be a priority for many mills, so the oil's carcinogenicity would gradually increase. It was not until 1945 that the industry was forced to use non-carcinogenic white oils. As you will read later, there are many parallels with the UK automotive industry, which in many areas did not conform to the 1945 standards of the now defunct Cotton industry until the 1980s.

1.5 Petrochemicals and mass production

The petrochemical industry was vastly expanded by the extremely rapid emergence of the new automotive industry over the period from 1900 to the Great War (1914–1918). Henry Ford (1863–1947) successfully adapted the assembly line concept used in the Chicago meat industry, and together with his durable Model T Ford design (you could reliably commute in one today, once you got used to the pedal arrangement), he was responsible for the phenomenal early growth of automobile manufacturing capacity. Indeed, although five million Model Ts had been produced up to 1921, this figure was actually doubled only three years later. By the 1930s, Ford's River Rouge complex at Dearborn in Michigan employed more than 100,000 workers. Such a growth stimulated other industries which were dependent on supplying the car and truck industry, which was well paid in comparison to most other manual labouring jobs, thus despite the repetitive nature of the assembly line, jobs with Ford were keenly sought.

The sheer scale and diversity of the different components of a motor vehicle spawned a vast engineering empire which involved subsidiary factories which employed various paint delivery systems, as well as metal casting, grinding, boring, plating, milling, stamping, broaching, heat-treating, welding and polishing processes. This meant that all these light engineering processes had their own often wasteful oil and lubricating processes, which ensured the machine tools operated efficiently. In addition, thousands of tonnes of different chemical solvents were involved in preparing (such as degreasing) metals for all these processes. Large amounts of component welding, cutting and stamping took place alongside the routine machine tool operation, as well as engine testing without rocker covers. All this created a dense mix of oil vapour, combustion and welding fumes which formed a thick fog inside the shop floors, which was an environment not dissimilar to the nineteenth-century cotton industry, where the fumes combined with machinery noise, heat and lack of ventilation. Indeed, workers' testaments from the UK and US car industries as late as the early 1980s described that the oil and fume mists were such that it was difficult to see more than a few yards. Given that very high oil mist levels in car factories before World War II resulted in workers suffering from bronchitis and other direct lung irritation–based complaints, it had been appreciated by plant managers even then that it was necessary to restrict atmospheric oil contamination. Gradually, the industry began to control the mists through better ventilation and more efficient machinery as the 1950s and 1960s progressed, although oil and fume mist levels were not by any means eliminated.

As with the cotton industry, the key danger of the mists was the carcinogenic nature of the oils used. In the United Kingdom, the automotive industry was slow to appreciate this risk, and it was not until the early 1960s that it belatedly realised that aromatic hydrocarbon content in a mineral oil was the chief determinant of its potential carcinogenicity. Unfortunately, as will be described in Chapter 4, mid-1960s recommendations that cutting fluids used to machine car components should not contain mineral oils with any aromatics, were not heeded. Automobile industry workers today often do not engender great sympathy in the United States and United Kingdom, partly because of historically poor labour relations and a reputation for militancy, allied to what was still in the 1970s and 1980s considerably higher pay than many other occupations. However, up to the 1980s, the available evidence and testimony suggest that it was not a pleasant industry to work in and it was resistant to lessons learned from other industries over issues related to toxic oils. This meant that metal cutting right into the late 1970s involved exposure to carcinogenic aromatic hydrocarbons, as well as to nitrosamines liberated from cutting fluid emulsions containing amine antioxidants. This translated into higher levels of cancers related to other industries. In a General Motors subsidiary factory at Coldwater Road near Flint, Michigan as late as 1980, several workers noticed that the mice in the plant were developing visible tumours, which they reported to their Union. Some mice were caught and tested, revealing that the tumours were cancerous. The metal-plating processes which the plant specialised in became outmoded with the advent of various plastic replacements and the plant was closed. However, it left a considerable number of ex-workers who had developed lung cancers at comparatively early ages.

The car industry has responded to these hazards in some ways that are akin to how armaments industries adapt to wartime, by changing manufacturing to reduce labour-intensive and expensive grinding, cutting and milling of components, in favour of stampings and mouldings which can be automated to the point where men are usually no longer in contact with toxic agents. Paint shops are fully automated and sealed, and volatile aromatic solvent paint bases have been replaced by safer and more environmentally friendly water-based systems. The industry remains profitable as although safety has been increased, costs have been reduced partly because fewer workers are often employed as a consequence. Car factories have evolved to the point that many manufacturers invite customers to watch their cars being assembled. However, as relatively new processes become established in the industry, such as the use of epoxy resins to bond metals, followed by some welding (weld bonding), this can create hazardous fumes which have not been fully investigated to date. In some factories, up to 50 different adhesives are used in the assembly process, and it has been reported that the famous 'new car smell' might be somewhat more problematic than was previously envisaged.

1.6 Aromatic amines: Tyres, dyes, explosives and cigarettes

The coal tar distilling business of the mid-nineteenth century gave birth to several industries as mentioned in section 1.4, mostly through a key discovery made by the English chemist, William Henry Perkin (1838–1907). Young Perkin was earmarked as a potential architect by his father, but became obsessed with chemistry when still a teenager. Indeed, the sheer ferocity of his interest in the subject led him to build a laboratory in his house, as he was too busy at college to pursue all the chemistry that interested him. Whilst trying to make a synthetic antimalarial, he treated aniline distilled from coal tar with the oxidising agent potassium dichromate and made a rather disgusting-looking black precipitate, which Perkin subsequently discovered was actually an effective purple or, as the French named it, 'mauve' dye. He then set about inventing the industrial process to make this dye in quantity and became the father of the aniline-derived dye industry, despite many authority figures insisting that he would never be able to scale up his inventions successfully. Perkin sold his factory in 1874 for a tidy sum, which allowed him to spend the rest of his life as what could be perhaps termed today as a postdoctoral dye researcher. He was by all accounts an extremely pleasant individual, hugely respected by his peers and who was devoted to his work and his family.

Aniline dyes were successful in the clothing, leather and many other industries due to the dye tending not to run and also that it would colour the surface of the item evenly and retain elements of the natural features of the cloth. As the dye industry became a large-scale employer, particularly in Germany, it became apparent that working in the industry could lead to developing bladder cancer. This was first reported in 1895, by the German surgeon Ludwig Rehn (1849–1930) [15], who investigated cases in a German aniline factory. With the beginning of the Great War in 1914, the German dye industry was turned over largely to explosives manufacture, and incidentally, their large watch and clock industry was given over to making timing mechanisms for explosive devices of various types. The difficulty in obtaining German-sourced dyes and the US entry into the war in 1917 led to the establishment of the industry in the United States by companies such as Du Pont (E. I. du Pont de Nemours and Company) in Wilmington, Delaware, and within a couple of decades, bladder cancer rates had dramatically increased in US dye workers in the Du Pont factories. By the late 1940s, it was established that rather than aniline itself, it was various aromatic amines linked to aniline processing which were responsible for the cancers, particularly β-naphthylamine (BNA) and benzidine. These agents and several other aromatic amines remain among the ever-growing list of chemicals and other agents which are accepted as human carcinogens [16]. From the early twentieth century, BNA was used in tyre manufacture as an antioxidant to slow the natural hardening and physical deterioration processes seen in automotive tyres, but its use was banned in the United Kingdom in 1949, and it was replaced by phenyl-BNA (PBNA). BNA continued to be manufactured around the world, such as in China and other developing countries and their bladder cancer incidences duly rose after the 20–30 years' cancer latency period elapsed. Whilst a perhaps small proportion (around 4–10%) of bladder cancer cases are probably linked to other polycyclic aromatics, such as benzopyrene, it has become apparent that most bladder cancers contracted in various industries are linked with BNA and benzidine derivatives, which were either used in chemical processes or were formed during combustion of petrochemicals, such as in coke ovens and in metal smelting.

It is useful to remember that although occupation is linked with bladder cancer, the major cause of the disease is actually tobacco smoking, although the specific chemical responsible remains BNA. As will be discussed in Chapter 4, these multiple sources of BNA and the possibility of its formation from supposedly safer substitutes can complicate the assessment of causation in cases of occupational bladder cancer.

1.7 Contemporaneous knowledge

So far in this brief introduction to occupational toxicity, a pattern can perhaps be discerned. An industry gradually emerges, using certain machinery, processes, work practices, chemicals and design of premises. This industry then becomes increasingly successful and powerful, through engaging whole communities in long hours of manual labour, which not only supports those communities, but makes certain individuals and their fellow investors incredibly rich and politically influential. Over time, it is noticed that the process of manufacture is associated with an abnormal morbidity and mortality in the workforce, and medical research is carried out on both the effects on the workers and basic research proceeds on the specific nature of the hazard. The knowledge of why the agent is toxic gradually surfaces in the scientific and medical press, which filters through to publications related to the industry and sometimes through to the local and national press. At some point during this process, which may last decades, the industry might take heed that its activities are causing mortality and morbidity, and it 'does the decent thing' by setting aside money to compensate the workers injured by the process and changing the activity and/or agent which is responsible for the problem.

Of course, this is far from an ideal situation, as it is clear that many workers will have been injured before action is taken, and their path to individual compensation is usually immeasurably more painful, expensive and protracted than those that might benefit from the first compensation initiative. Many industries over the last two centuries have followed a similar course to that described above, as often the nature of the specific mechanisms whereby a chemical or industrial process injures an individual chronically was simply not known until the sheer scale of the process or the chemical usage for a considerable period of time reveals the risk and the mechanism is determined by medical and scientific personnel. Indeed, a key factor in all claims for compensation from an employer or more likely, their insurance company, is linked to 'contemporaneous knowledge'. Should the employer have known that the agent was a hazard at the time the workers were exposed and if they did know, then why did they not take steps to protect them from the hazard? In real life, there are many shades of employer culpability, and to be fair, workers themselves can be notoriously resistant to complying with Health and Safety measures. In addition, a charitable view is often taken, where there can be significant lag-times between large and cumbersome organisations 'digesting' information which is ascribed to a combination of internal rigidity and poor communication.

1.8 The pursuit of truth

It is easy for us today in the developed world to pass withering judgement on the horrors of our industrial past, without perhaps considering the activities of an industry in the context of the standards which were held at the time. Today, it is much easier to champion the emancipation of illegal child labourers in the United Kingdom, than, say in India, China or Vietnam. As we saw earlier, the protracted resistance to the banning of child chimney sweeps in the United Kingdom was probably partly a result of the somewhat schizophrenic early Victorian attitude to children, where childhood could be idolised, whilst children were routinely maltreated. In Germany, the work of Johann Frank (1745–1821) and later in England of Thackrah in 1832 [17] as well as Chadwick a decade later [18] not only revealed the suffering of many in various trades which were hugely injurious to health, but also demanded passionately that this situation be changed in direct terms. These authors and many others in the industrialised nations of the nineteenth century drew attention to the fact that life expectancy was strongly linked to social class, and alongside deprivation and poor living standards, occupation was a powerful influence on mortality and morbidity.

Changes in social attitudes had to occur before there could be recognition of workers' rights, and this process was and remains agonisingly slow. However, many industries carried on exposing their workers to conditions which were unacceptable even by the standards of the time. In the United Kingdom today, whilst we assume we live in a progressive and just society, situations emerge where a group of individuals are exposed to a sustained injustice, which is only confronted once a courageous individual has exposed the perpetrators to public opprobrium. However, it has almost become a cliché in real life, cinematic and televisual entertainment that this individual was probably actually sent to investigate the problem, but often meets determined resistance from powerful and influential quarters, sometimes even from those who entrusted them with their mission in the first place. Likewise in occupational medicine, institutional resistance to investigation and clarity is often to be expected, and stratagems must be evolved to determine the truth to help the worker. As far back as 1848, the Prussian doctor Rudolf Virchow lost his office, job and salary for revealing the extent of the social depravation in Silesian miners when he was actually sent to investigate a medical emergency in the area. Even into the mid-twentieth century, workers in industrialised countries who reported occupationally linked disease risked being regarded as lazy or feckless, and even talking to a healthcare professional could lead to dismissal. Companies and organisations refused to release details of their workers' health and obstructed anyone who sought such information. Occupational medical pioneers in the United States such as Alice Hamilton (1869–1970) could only build a picture of the extent of lead poisoning in many industries through what was termed 'shoe-leather epidemiology' [19]. This involved tirelessly tracking down workers' records and persuading individuals in numerous industries over many years to report their symptoms and working practices which caused their ill-health. Nearly a century later, Figueroa and Weiss [20] employed similar techniques to reveal the carcinogenicity of bischloromethyl-ether in spite of the determined resistance of the chemical industry.

Sadly, there remain many examples of employers who did know of the hazards, yet chose not to protect those at risk. Worse still, there were many whole industries which were collectively aware of the devastating consequences for their workers of handling certain agents, and they were not only resistant to providing protective equipment, but they were also extremely active in escaping their liabilities and responsibility for their worker's plight. The next sections recount a brief history of three industries which perhaps typify this somewhat extreme situation; the early twentieth-century radium dial industry, the asbestos business and, of course, the hat industry.

1.9 The 'Mad Hatter'

Lewis Carroll's depiction of a somewhat bizarre milliner in *Alice in Wonderland* (1865) has now passed into popular culture as a terrible example of occupational toxicity related to the use of mercury to treat felt. The truth could well be more complex, as the book was published in a period where it has been latterly argued that there was actually little common perception of hat making as particularly dangerous, despite some contemporary medical reports of mercury poisoning associated with handling hat making materials. Indeed, it is said that Carroll's inspiration may have been a slightly unhinged but creative individual known as Theophilus Carter, a top-hatted Oxford furniture dealer who apparently invented an 'alarm clock bed' which woke the sleeper by physically turfing them onto floor. This inspired invention could yet find a lucrative online market today with the parents of particularly indolent teenagers. It is believed now that the phrases 'mad as a hatter' or 'mad as a March hare' pre-dated *Alice in Wonderland* by several decades. It appears that the story of how mercury became involved in the hat business is also somewhat confused and convoluted.

Until the end of the seventeenth century, hats were made from various woven fibres, but the use of fairly poor-quality animal skins (particularly rabbit) to make hat felt began in France and necessitated some processing to make the material resistant to rotting, by altering the protein structure as well as firstly removing the fur or hair from the hides. The leather industry used various substances including urine to remove hair from the hide, and the emerging hat industry followed a similar practice, until legend has it that the urine of a worker under mercury treatment for venereal disease had the best results. This was known to the French as the *secretage* and the industry was dominated by Huguenots, who were effectively hounded out of France after the 1685 Edict of Fontainebleau withdrew their freedom of religion. Hence, they migrated to England, along with their expertise in hat-making. The *secretage* involved using mercury nitrate to shrink and lift the fur off the hide. The fur would turn orange, giving the name of 'carroting' to the process [21], which seemed to die out after the end of the eighteenth century in England, only to resume around the 1840s.

The epicentre in North America of the hat industry from the early eighteenth century was Danbury in Connecticut, where beaver was first used, and interestingly, their hides did not require mercury to treat them to make high-quality felt. However, as with the North American Bison, over-hunting virtually wiped the beaver out, so rabbit and other small animals were drawn into the highly profitable Danbury operation, and at its peak, mercury nitrate became an essential of the processing of more than five million hats per year [22]. The hat industry in the United States was associated with debilitating toxicity from as early as the 1830s and from the 1860s all the way to the 1920s; a succession of medical reports drew attention to the damage mercury caused to hatters' health. Little was done to prevent it, by either protecting the workers or by seeking alternative processing materials.

As early as 1874, a method appeared to replace mercury and towards the end of the nineteenth century, there were several more methods available [23, 24]. However, as with the master chimney sweeps, the industry was highly resistant to change, and it carried on using mercury to the point that it had to be banned by the US Government in December 1941, although this initiative may have owed more to the coming need for mercury in the munitions industry, rather than concern for workers. Even today, the legacy of mercury use is the extremely high environmental mercury pollution in areas where the hat industry flourished, such as Danbury [22].

The effects of mercury on those who worked in the industry were appalling. Many developed unpleasant central nervous system and peripheral effects, including a staggering gait, severe tremors and often extreme irritability with unpredictable behaviour which must have made them impossible to live with. Those most affected also suffered from visual problems, drooling and even hallucinations. The 'shakes' were sometimes even identified with a particular area where the hat industry was very large, entering the local language as the 'Danbury Shakes'. In the United Kingdom, a report on a worker who used mercury nitrate to process animal hides who was admitted to Guy's Hospital with mercury poisoning in 1863 is interesting, as it locates the use of mercury in England from the end of the 1850s, as the individual had only been working with the toxin for four years. This also has to be seen in the context of mercury toxicity, as neither the metal vapour itself nor an aerosol which contains mercury ions is even the most toxic form of the metal. Organo-mercurials, such as methyl mercury, are especially neurotoxic, as they are lipophilic (fat soluble) enough to penetrate the blood brain barrier. This, combined with the relatively short period of exposure prior to debilitating symptoms, suggests that the scale of daily worker exposure to mercury in the hat industry must have been phenomenal. Whilst mercury toxicity was made a notifiable disease as early as 1899 in Britain, even as late as the 1930s, several studies failed to link clinical symptoms of mercury poisoning with urinary metal levels, probably due to crude analysis techniques. Eventually, a group in Milan published a study in 1953 which showed that more than a sixth of workers in the industry showed mercury poisoning. Ironically, not so long after mercury use was banned in the industry, changes in fashion virtually eliminated the felt-based hat industry after the 1960s.

As mercury usage receded in the moribund hat industry, the metal found a use as a catalyst in the formation of acetaldehyde, a key component in plastics manufacture. Methyl mercury was a by-product of this process and the Chisso Corporation dumped up to 150 tonnes of this potent neurotoxin and teratogen into Minamata Bay in southern Japan from 1932 to 1968. The ensuing human and environmental catastrophe cost more than 1700 lives and damaged the health of two million people [25]. There was so much mercury present in the sludge of the factory's wastewater canal, that it was commercially viable for the Chisso corporation to recover, which they duly did. The clean-up operation cost nearly $US400 million and took 14 years, and the residents of the bay continue to suffer and legal action has not yet been resolved. Another organo-mercurial agent, phenyl mercuric acetate, was used in processes which exploited its antifungal effects, such as in latex paint manufacture (until 1990) and as a seed dressing. It was also used to catalyse the curing of polyethylene flexible flooring, which was used in thousands of school gymnasia from the 1950s to the 1970s [26].

Although many countries have banned mercury usage as a pesticide, it is still used to preserve vaccines, in dental amalgams and particularly destructively, in small-scale gold mining. In this latter application, although systems have been developed to recycle the metal and reduce environmental damage, there remains widespread ignorance amongst workers handling this metal, as to its severe impact on health [27].

1.10 The 'Radium Girls'

Whilst this book is concerned with the evaluation of causation linked with occupational toxins such as metals or petrochemicals, no brief history of occupational toxicity is complete without reference to one of the most poignant occupationally linked tragedies, that of the 'Radium Girls'. Today many of us have watches, mobile phones or various electronic reading platforms which allow perusal of life's latest fascinating developments in total darkness and probably even underwater, for essentially unlimited time. Towards the end of the Great War, the idea of soldiers being able to read a watch or an instrument panel at night was a remarkable innovation, and it was achieved through a paint called 'Undark', which was a mix of radium and zinc sulphide, where the alpha and beta particles from the radium would cause the sulphide to emit a faint glow. This innovation was the product of an ex-laboratory assistant of Thomas Edison, William Joseph Hammer (1858–1934), who combined several careers as a soldier, inventor and tireless promoter of all things related to radium. However, 'successful businessman' was not part of his portfolio, as he did not patent his idea, which by 1920 had led to more than four million clocks and watches produced with radium paint dials. The War had propelled radium-sourced luminous paint towards its vast market, and the Radium Luminous Material Corporation was the first organisation to exploit this idea on a large scale. They became the US Radium Corporation and by the early 1920s, the young ladies in their factory in New Jersey were trained to paint numerals on watch dials by instructors, who showed them how to use their lips to make a fine point on the brush to allow the accurate formation of certain awkward numbers, such as 8, 2, 3 and 6. The instructors in the watch factories would consume the radium paint during the demonstration, somewhat eerily echoed 40 years later in the Vietnam-era news footage of a US Air Force Officer drinking a cup of Agent Orange (see Chapter 5) out of an aircraft tank to demonstrate to his men that it was harmless.

Whilst the women in the factories became massively contaminated with radium and even sometimes used it to paint their nails and even their teeth with it to impress the unwary in the dark, it seems the owners of the factory and their senior personnel were well aware of the toxicity of their product, which is not surprising, as US Radium was started by medical doctors. The Company scientists actually took the same precautions we take today to shield themselves from the danger. The 'Radium Girls' gradually became sick, as the metal mimicked calcium and accumulated in their bones, particularly their jaws; indeed, their terrible injuries were first recognised by a dentist, Theodore Blum [28]. US Radium, in their efforts to escape responsibility for this tragedy, acted in a way that can only be described as stomach churning, with deliberate and persistent attempts to falsify reports and to draw out the court process, knowing that the women were unlikely to survive long enough to collect much compensation. Indeed, during the court case, some of the women did not have the strength to move their arms enough to take the oath. Only a public outcry allowed them any real financial settlement at all, as the workers were not members of a union and had to organise their cases themselves [29]. A medical report described how contaminated many of the workers were, with many having been exposed to thousands of times the recommended safe dose of radiation. Their clothes and bodies were heavily contaminated to the point of luminosity, as indeed was the discoverer of radium herself, Marie Curie. To this day, the double Nobel Prize winner's domestic cookbook is too radioactive to read without protective equipment. There were many thousands of women employed in various factories using radium paint, and it is unknown how many died prematurely from its use.

1.11   Asbestos

Perhaps the best known and documented of the various industries which are known to be purveyors of disability and premature death is the Asbestos Industry. Interestingly, the properties of these silicate mineral fibres have been known since antiquity, with several accounts in existence of various potentates impressing their guests by cleaning their asbestos tableware by throwing it on the fire, presumably with the ancient equivalent of a theatrical flourish and a smug visage. Pliny left an account of these fibres' many uses, and the Chinese were mining it in quantity by the thirteenth century. The great Georgius Agricola investigated it, partly and somewhat eccentrically, by describing its taste. By the mid-twentieth century, it had found its way into millions of products, ranging from cigarette filters (obviously), brake linings and clutches, through to myriad lagging and building products. Indeed, it has been possible to have a fireproof suit made since 1820.

There are six fibre types recognised as asbestos, with only three ever being produced in quantity. The hardest and straightest fibres are amosite (brown asbestos) and crocidolite (blue asbestos), and these have long been perceived as the most dangerous. They damage the lung because they cannot essentially be removed once they reach the alveoli, and through a combination of the creation of active reactive oxygen species and immunologically mediated damage, they can cause either/or the destruction of the lungs by inflammatory disease (asbestosis) or malignancy, particularly mesothelioma. This condition has killed many hundreds of thousands around the world, as well as the Hollywood star Steve McQueen (1930–1980), one of the protagonists in what is arguably cinema's premier car chase [30]. The vast majority of asbestos used was chrysotile (white asbestos), whose softer, snake-like fibres were believed to be less hazardous than the blue or brown variants. However, in practice, all manifestations of this mineral are toxic, carcinogenic and are unsafe at any level.

Whilst world consumption peaked in 1973 [31], the toxicity of these mineral fibres was first reported 75 years previously by a UK Factory Inspector, Lucy Deane. She and her colleagues made the link between the 'glass-like jagged nature' of the microscopic appearance of the fibres and their 'evil effects' [32]. Soon after, a Charing Cross Hospital doctor, H. Montague Murray, examined an asbestos worker and found severe pulmonary fibrosis. After the man's subsequent demise, Murray testified at a Compensation Committee that he found asbestos fibres in the patient's lungs and that they were the major cause of his death. The man had worked in a 'carding room' and told the doctor that of the 10 people who had worked with him in that room, he was the only survivor [33].

Over the next few years, progress in exploring asbestos's lethality was slow, although as early as 1918, it was impossible for asbestos workers to obtain life insurance from some companies in the United States. It was not until 1931 that regulations appeared in the United Kingdom to safeguard workers from the hazards of the mineral and in 1932, a report from the Inspector of Factories recognised asbestos's role in asbestosis. Incredibly, despite a series of official medical reports in the United Kingdom over the 1950s and 1960s damning the mineral, blue asbestos was only banned in 1985. I remember the 1982 Yorkshire Television documentary on those who worked in Cape Insulation Limited's Acre Mill in Hebden Bridge in Yorkshire, UK, from 1939 to 1970. The debilitation and hopelessness of the workers was appalling to see. Forty-five years after the Mill was closed, the Company eventually did establish a fund to compensate ex-workers, although it was estimated that more than 750 ex-workers had died from asbestos-related illnesses by 2003. This is all the more remarkable, as at its peak, the factory employed only 580 people. It was apparent that unlike other industrial diseases, where only certain individuals might be susceptible to the effects of handling a product, it appears that like mercury and radium, everyone is susceptible to asbestos. The mineral, almost entirely as chrysotile, is still mined around the world and remains in use in considerable quantity. Indeed, the focus of its production and usage has shifted dramatically over the past few decades to developing economies, primarily China,

India, Russia and Brazil, which account for 66% of current world production. Even in the developed world, asbestos may well be probably part of a wall or lagging a pipe, perhaps even not too far from where you are sitting now. However, as long as you can resist the urge to bore holes in the wall or sand the pipe down, it is highly unlikely that you will ever suffer any health impact from asbestos, as it almost exclusively affected those that worked with it. The asbestos industry in general is a byword for its reluctance to acknowledge its culpability in its workers' suffering, and as an industry, it could be justly described by the famous phrase 'the unacceptable face of capitalism'. It is still extremely active in protecting its interests [34], and it effectively 'owns' enough scientists to fight its corner, rather like a malevolent and loathsome infection. Asbestos is by a large margin, the worst occupational toxin ever [35] and its devastating health and financial impact will continue for many decades to come. Many would say that asbestos is now probably the most hated substance on the planet.

1.12   Occupational toxicity: Medicine and science

Occupational medicine ideally should be focussed in the prevention of mortality and morbidity, through enforcement of basic principles of industrial hygiene, which are in turn informed by medical and scientific principles which describe the nature of the hazard and the steps required to make it safe to work with. So in a perfect world, a new manufacturing process should be examined in detail by representatives of the manufacturing process, as well as scientists and medical personnel to uncover any risks to worker safety. Appropriate measures can then be devised and incorporated into the process which ensures that workers are fully protected, before the process is scaled up and begins in earnest. As has been described earlier, too often, the process of occupational medicine is retrospective and begins with ignorance, where doctors meet a set of symptoms with which they are unfamiliar and may not at first follow Ramazzini's exhortation to ask about occupation. In the case of 'Phossy Jaw' and also beryllium poisoning, many workers in the safety match and mining industries suffered from these diseases and doctors had very little, if any, worthwhile knowledge of these conditions, and medical training does not often explore occupational medicine in any depth [19]. Hence, many cases of occupational health damage require a team of experts to investigate and ultimately facilitate the victim's legitimate claim for compensation. Medical examination should initially record the victim's symptoms, and if the doctor is familiar with the industry and its impact on health, he or she can sometimes associate these with the industry. However, this is often not enough to ascribe causation, as many toxic effects can be mimicked by other diseases which are acquired through other means. It is now accepted that 'causation', that is, exactly how the toxin impacted the patient and led to their present condition, should be investigated for a specific case by an individual who has experience in either (sometimes both) the medical or scientific aspects of the toxin or disease.

Whilst there are many examples of expert testimony which have highlighted the dangers to workers, such as the work of von Volkmann for tar distillers and Alice Hamilton for many other trades, experts can sometimes be less than truthful, as we have seen in the Asbestos industry particularly, usually due to company or government pressure. At the other extreme, US Radium's first attempt at 'expert testimony' involved using their own toxicologist under blatantly false pretences, to certify that a transparently sick individual was healthy. When they did ask for an external expert report from the Harvard physiology professor, Cecil Drinker, they were very unhappy with its damning contents and falsified it. Alice Hamilton encouraged Drinker to publish his report which he did, even though the exceedingly wealthy and well-connected US Radium threatened legal action.

The prospect of litigation is daunting to anyone, and the behaviour of an organisation in this context is often related to the perception of ownership of the intellectual property of the report. If an organisation funds a report, it can believe that it has absolute legal control of the information unearthed [19]. Therefore, if this report is published without authorisation, the organisation may well have the means and the will to pursue the expert legally to enforce its position. Various laws, particularly UK libel law, can lend themselves relatively easily to the pursuit of individuals by powerful organisations, and the sheer expense of the process can bankrupt the individual, their supporters and even their publishers. In the United Kingdom, the key stage appears to be whether a statement or statements are viewed as allegations of 'fair comment' or 'fact'. 'Fair comment' may not be a problem, but if a statement is viewed by a judge as an 'allegation of fact', then this requires the defendant (the individual who made the allegation), rather than the claimant (the organisation), to prove the accuracy of their statements, so it pays to be extremely careful over the wording of an expert report [36], and it is perhaps not surprising that many large corporations and government-related organisations have been able to intimidate scientists and medical personnel. Many years ago, I contributed some comments over the health risks concerned with the process of extracting a particular metal in a substantial local facility to a journalist who published a decidedly inflammatory article in the local free press on the subject quoting my comments. The facility managing director almost immediately telephoned me in what can only be described as a Caledonian Fury and demanded that we should meet at the University to discuss how I was 'endangering 600 people's livelihoods'. I agreed to meet him in the presence of my then line manager and the managing director insisted aggressively that I recant my statements. He then dramatically produced a prepared statement that I was to sign to the effect that I was withdrawing my comments. I pointed out that I had merely quoted journal articles that were in the public domain and I produced some copies for his perusal, which he neglected to accept. He then departed in high dudgeon, emitting various dark legal threats. The statement was sent to me again in the post some days later, and I returned it unsigned, restating my position. The managing director then contacted the Vice-Chancellor of my University on more than one occasion and demanded that I should be sacked; the Vice-Chancellor eventually explained to him in apparently direct terms that no action would be taken against me and perhaps he should cease and desist, which brought the matter to a close.

In my case, I was supported fully by my institution; however, other scientists have not enjoyed such backing and have been put under unbearable pressure by various industries, the media, government and other organisations, sometimes with tragic consequences.

1.13   Health and safety today

Whilst it is sometimes fashionable to criticise Health and Safety organisations for overzealous enforcement of various legislation, in the light of even this brief history of occupational toxicity, such zeal is not necessarily a bad thing. In the developed world at least, the tragically long delays between the identification of a toxin's potential role in human morbidity and mortality should now be a thing of the past, as most organisations have access to the latest research and various techniques for monitoring workers' health, to ensure that the use of hazardous agents is fully investigated and that workers health is of paramount importance, if only for financial reasons. However, there remain many organisations, both large and small, which refuse to acknowledge their duty of care to their workforce and whilst many believe that this no longer occurs in developed countries and is now exclusively the part of so-called third-world sweatshops in various eastern boom economies, some of the cases described in this book will hopefully disabuse them of this impression. There remain vulnerable groups of workers in developed countries who can be exploited and exposed to hazardous agents, either through language difficulties or ignorance. In developing countries, the hunger for wealth generation and employment, coupled with a ruthless exploitative 'ethic' which would have impressed many nineteenth-century stove pipe-hatted capitalists, can lead to horrifying worker morbidity and mortality. Indeed, as we will see in Chapter 6, since many of the products of eastern economies are not even safe for the user, so it is sobering to wonder how they are manufactured and under what conditions. Some workers have even smuggled out letters asking for help hidden in their products, to be discovered by consumers overseas [37]. Perhaps more than ever, experts in their scientific and medical fields are needed to engage with cases where their knowledge may be of benefit to an individual, or individuals, who have been harmed by their occupation.

References

1. Debus AG. World Who's Who in Science: A Biographical Dictionary of Notable Scientists from Antiquity to the Present. Marquis, Chicago, 1968.
2. Waldron HA. Lead poisoning in the ancient world. Med Hist. 17, 391–399, 1973.
3. Aitchison L. A History of Metals, vol. 1. Interscience Pub., London, p 43, 1960.
4. Agricola Georgius; De Re Metallica .... http://www.gutenberg.org/files/38015/38015-h/38015-h.htm. Gutenberg ebook; (accessed March 2013).

5. Borzelleca JF. Paracelsus: herald of modern toxicology. Toxicol Sci. 53, 2–4, 2000.
6. Grzesik JP, Sokal JA. Occupational Hygiene and Health Care in Polish Coal Mines. Institute of Occupational Medicine and Environmental Health Sosnowiec, Sosnowiec, pp 1–14, 2003.
7. Nelson G et al. Three decades of silicosis: disease trends at autopsy in South African gold miners. Environ Health Perspect. 118, 421–426, 2010.
8. Lenin VI. A great technical achievement. Pravda, April 21, p 91, 1913.
9. Franco G, Franco F. Bernardino Ramazzini: the father of occupational medicine. Am J Public Health. 91, 1382, 2001.
10. Hunter D. The Diseases of Occupations. English University Press, London, 1975.
11. Pott P. Chirurgical Observations Relative to the Cataract, the Polypus of the Nose, the Cancer of the Scrotum, the Different Kinds of Ruptures, and the Mortification of the Toes and Feet. Hawes, Clarke & Collins, London, 7–13, 1775.
12. von Volkmann R. Beitrage sur Chirurgie. Breitkopf und Hartel, Leipzig, p 370, 1875.
13. Yamagiwa K, Ichikawa K. Experimental study of the pathogenesis of carcinoma. J Cancer Res. 3, 1–29, 1918.
14. Twort CC, Twort JM. Induction of cancer by cracked mineral oils. Lancet. 2, 1226–1228, 1935.
15. Rehn L. Blasengeschuwulste bei Fuchsin-Arbeitern Arch Klin Chir. 50, 588–600, 1895.
16. NTP. Report on Carcinogens, 12th edition. Research Triangle Park: U.S. Department of Health and Human Services, Public Health Service, National Toxicology Program, 499 pp, 2011. http://ntp.niehs.nih.gov/ntp/roc/twelfth/roc12.pdf (accessed on 11 November 2013).
17. Thackrah CT. The Effects of the Principal Arts, Trades and Professions, and of Civic States and Habits of Living, on Health and Longevity, with Suggestions for the Removal of Many of the Agents which Produce Disease and Threaten the Duration of Life, 2nd edition. Longman, London, 1832. Cited in Sigerist (1960), 54–55.
18. Chadwick E. The Sanitary Condition of the Labouring Population of Great Britain. Edinburgh University Press, Edinburgh, 1842, reprinted 1965.
19. Abrams HK. A short history of occupational health. Adv Mod Environ Toxicol. 22, 33–71, 1994.
20. Figueroa WG, Weiss W. Lung cancer in chloromethyl ether workers. N Engl J Med. 288, 1096–1097, 1973.
21. Goldwater LJ. The hat industry. In: Mercury; A History of Quicksilver. New York Press, New York, 1965.
22. Van Patten P. The Mad Hatter Mercury Mystery. Wrack Lines. Paper 24, 2002. http://digitalcommons.uconn.edu/wracklines/24 (accessed on 11 November 2013).
23. Von Delpech HA. Method of preparing the fur of rabbits and hares for the manufacture of felt without the use of mercury. J Chem Soc. Abstract. 27, 99, 1874.
24. Dargelos MJA. Process of Preparing Animal-Hairs for Felting. U.S. Patent 390, 348, 2 October 1888.
25. McCurry J. Japan remembers Minamata. Lancet. 367(9505), 99–100, 2006.
26. Beaulieu HJ et al. Phenyl mercuric acetate (PMA): mercury-bearing flexible gymnasium floors in schools – evaluation of hazards and controlled abatement. J Occup Environ Hyg. 5, 360–366, 2008.

27. Jonsson JB et al. Toxic mercury versus appropriate technology: artisanal gold miners' retort aversion. Res Policy. 38, 60–67, 2013.
28. Mullner R. Deadly Glow: The Radium Dial Worker Tragedy. American Public Health Association, Washington, DC, 1989.
29. Rosner D, Markowitz G. Dying for Work. Indiana University Press, Bloomington, 53–63, 208, 221, 1987.
30. McQueen TS, Bisset WJF, Vaughn Dr RF in 'Bullitt'; Dir. Peter Yates, Warner Bros. Seven Arts, 113 min, October 1968.
31. Alleman JE, Mossman BT. Asbestos revisited. Sci Am. 277, 70–75, 1997.
32. Deane L. 1899. Report on the health of workers in asbestos and other dusty trades. In HM Chief Inspector of Factories and Workshops, Annual Report for 1898. London: HMSO, 171–172.
33. Murray HM. 1906. Departmental Committee on Compensation for Industrial Diseases, 1907, Minutes of Evidence. London: HMSO, 127.
34. Holmes D. IARC in the dock over ties with asbestos industry. Lancet. 381(9864): 359–361, 2013.
35. Peto J. The European mesothelioma epidemic. Brit J Cancer 79, 666–672, 1999.
36. Adams S. Simon Singh wins key battle in alternative medicine libel case, 2010. www.telegraph.co.uk/health/healthnews/7544666/Simon-Singh-wins-key-battle-in-alternative-medicine-libel-case.html# (accessed on 11 November 2013).
37. Cavaliere V. Oregon woman finds letter in sealed toy box, purportedly from Chinese worker in a labour camp pleading for help, 2012. http://www.nydailynews.com/news/national/toy-box-letter-china-labor-camp-article-1.1228302 (accessed on 11 November 2013).

2

The expert report process in legal context

2.1 The would-be claimant's initial position

Millions of workers around the world handle toxic or hazardous materials over their professional lives and a substantial minority will develop serious disease related to their work. Such a disease might have been developing for many years with or sometimes without the individual's knowledge. The condition may be acute or chronic, resulting in outcomes ranging from complete or partial recovery, through to lifelong debilitation and premature death. Work-related ill-health can strike at any time in life and may well prevent an individual from working for a period of time. If this occurs when the individual is relatively young, then if they recover from their condition and it is clear that the working process was responsible for their problems, they may at best be able to work for the same employer using a different process. Alternatively, they may lose their job and be unable to work for some time until they recover. In addition, they may be effectively forced out of a position or craft where they have considerable experience and have more than likely devoted many years to acquiring specific skills associated with the work. Aside from the financial consequences of a loss of skilled livelihood, there is also the psychological impact, where an individual mourns the loss of a craft that meant a great deal to them in terms of status and work satisfaction and they face either a gruelling period of retraining or the prospect of the remainder of their working lives spent in a job from which they derive little or no satisfaction. Irrespective of whether the individual recovers, they will be aware that their occupation caused their ill-health, and they may wish to seek redress for the injury they received.

However, in many other cases, occupationally related disease strikes comparatively late in working life and when the individual becomes too incapacitated to work, it is unlikely they will find other employment even if they recovered. In yet other scenarios, the individual might have long left the trade that led to the problem, but is then prevented from pursuing an alternative career due to the injuries caused by the first trade. In any case, many of the most serious chronic occupational diseases

Expert Report Writing in Toxicology: Forensic, Scientific and Legal Aspects,
First Edition. Michael D. Coleman.
© 2014 John Wiley & Sons, Ltd. Published 2014 by John Wiley & Sons, Ltd.

strike in the final years of a working life or even in the first years of retirement, when the individual is looking forward to spending time with their family. Instead, what remains of their lives can be spent in a complex, stressful and ultimately futile rear-guard action against the consequences of the employment choices of their youth.

Of course, serious conditions such as severe respiratory damage or various can-cers can be caused by combinations of many factors aside from occupation, not least smoking, diet, lifestyle choices and genetic predispositions. Therefore, unless the individual worked for an industry notoriously linked with their condition and has therefore known friends and work colleagues to suffer the same condition, the first reaction of the medical help sought is to treat the condition, rather than neces-sarily immediately ascribe causation. If a healthcare professional treating the indi-vidual follows Ramazzini's exhortation to enquire after occupation and makes a link between occupation and disease, this may be the first inkling the individual might have that his or her condition is not just a random 'bad luck' event. This may be linked to other cases the professional has seen or perhaps his or her awareness of the reputation an industry has developed. In the absence of a medical perspective on the causation of the individual's condition, the vast repository of information on the World Wide Web has allowed individuals to research the condition themselves and find large amounts of relevant information which they may or may not understand or appreciate. Other important sources of information are local bodies which pro-vide invaluable and unflagging advice, support and information to workers about occupationally induced ill-health; a short list of some of these organisations in the United Kingdom appears at the end of this chapter [1–4].

Once the patient believes that their injury might be linked to their former occupa-tion, their best plan is to consult their General Practitioner and enlist their support, who could arrange a referral to an Occupational Health Advisor. This professional can provide relevant information to assist with the individual's second most press-ing problem after their medical condition, which may well be how to support themselves and any dependants financially.

2.2   Industrial injuries disablement benefit

If the individual is debilitated by occupational disease, they may have had to retire considerably earlier than they anticipated, and most pension schemes pay out noticeably less to those who retire in their 50s compared with those who worked to their 60s. In addition, the individual's medical condition may require extra financial support, directed at activities which improve quality of life. Hence, if the individual has a strong suspicion that their condition is work related, it is worthwhile entering the process whereby they apply to the Department of Work and Pensions (DWP) for Industrial Injuries Disablement Benefit [5], which is an occupational injury–linked pension. Sadly, awareness of this pathway is poor amongst the people who should be benefiting from it. Essentially, the DWP administers a process whereby the Industrial Injuries Advisory Council stipulates which work-related diseases are 'prescribed'. Whilst there are over 70 diseases listed as prescribed [5], if an individual is suffering from a condition that they believe is work related and it is not on the list of prescribed diseases, then any application for benefit will be turned down. The system of prescribed diseases lists them as 'A' related to physical causes, such as repetitive strain, housemaid's knee or deafness; 'B' which is linked with biological causes, such as various gruesome infections sustained from working with sewage and/or animals; 'C' stands for chemical causes, which includes various organ damage related to chemical exposure and finally 'D' which describes other conditions, which can range from allergies, to lung cancers and emphysema.

In practice, the claimant fills in the supplied DWP form and the questions posed are effectively the same questions that a solicitor will ask, if the claimant wishes to start legal proceedings against their employer. The questions should establish the veracity of the claim, which will include determining whether the claimant's disease is prescribed, its date of onset and if it can be linked with the claimant's employment and his specific duties. A 'diagnosis question' is posed, which is intended to establish the details of the affliction, as well as the degree of impairment the individual is suffering. If the claim is successful, benefit is scaled according to the DWP's perception of the impairment.

After establishing the basics, such as whether the individual actually worked for the employer in question, the claimant is examined by doctors and then a decision is taken by a 'decision maker'. The terms of the regulations can be extremely narrow, and if, for example, an individual claims with bladder cancer, then they will only succeed if they can prove that they were exposed to at least one or other of the list of chemicals in section C23 of Appendix 1 of the DWP List of diseases covered by Industrial Injuries Disablement Benefit. In practice, virtually all these agents have been long banned or are no longer part of industrial processes. In any case, few individuals will be able to remember which specific chemicals they used a decade or in some cases three decades or more in the past. Whilst statistically, it is glaringly obvious that it is highly unlikely that a female non-smoker would develop bladder cancer, if such a situation did present itself to this system, then unless the claimant could prove that they were exposed to the chemicals listed in C23, then their claim would fail. The system can be appealed, usually to a panel of one or two medical experts and a chairperson. However, unless more information can be presented, the situation is unlikely to change. Hence, an individual might find they are unable to claim Industrial Injury Benefit, unable to work, in receipt of an inadequate pension and in possession of a powerful sense of injustice. Their only recourse will then be to approach a solicitor with a view to instituting proceedings against their employer.

2.3   The legal process: First steps

As a would-be claimant, probably the first investigations should take place in one's nearest city or town, to find law partnerships that specialise in occupational claims. This can make a significant difference to how quickly the claim can progress, as not all high-street solicitors have gathered sufficient expertise to judge whether a claim of this type has any real prospects of reaching court. Specialist occupational claim law partnerships are likely to be found in larger cities, and whilst this is a disadvantage in terms of travel and inconvenience, it is more than worthwhile in providing a good start to the legal process. Law firms which handle such claims on a daily basis have the appropriate experience, as well as the contact details of a number of experts of medical and scientific background who can assist with investigating the case. Indeed, in the 1990s, the then Legal Aid Board awarded block contracts to specialist law firms to handle group claims made on common areas such as organophosphates. This was because the cases involved similar injuries, causations and even defendants. It is also important that the would-be claimant looks at the Civil Procedure Rules, which are to be found on the Ministry of Justice website [6]. There is a very large amount of detailed guidance set out on this site, alongside the appropriate forms to be submitted as part of the case, so the claimant can see how the whole process works.

2.4   Legal advice: Who pays?

It is strongly recommended by the Civil Procedure Rules that appropriate legal advice should be taken before embarking on any legal quest and of course such specialised advice is expensive. To mount a case, the solicitor's initial investigations must be funded, as well as in due course other direct costs such as the commissioning of expert reports from relevantly qualified medical and scientific personnel. In addition, there will be the various costs incurred through the first 'pre-action' protocols (Section 2.6) which are required to be applied before any case comes to court.

In the past, the Legal Aid process would often fund civil proceedings, but today there is a perception that Legal Aid is now only available to the mega-rich and the destitute, with pretty much nobody in between. This is not entirely true, and eligibility for Legal Aid is set out by the Legal Aid Agency (LAA), which replaced the Legal Services Commission in April 2013 [7]. In essence, the decision is made using three sets of criteria. Firstly, what type of legal proceedings are involved, secondly, the claimants earnings and assets, followed by thirdly, whether they have a realistic chance of victory, which might recover costs. In terms of the proceedings involved, there are several types of claim that are ineligible, such as personal injury for example, but occupational health claims are likely to be eligible. Financial eligibility will be decided upon using information on disposable income, cash, property and other assets of the claimant, as well as their partners' assets. As of 2013, for example, if you earn (or receive) less than £12,475 per annum, then you will be eligible for Legal Aid [7], whilst a monthly income of more than £2657 per month (more depending on how many children you have) or if you have more than £8000 in cash means that you will not be considered. Even if you are between these limits, the LAA may not necessarily agree to fund the case. If the LAA decide in your favour, the claimant might still have to pay towards the case in terms of a lump sum, or a charge based on their monthly income, or more usually, a 'statutory charge' which is basically taken from the claimant's winnings if the case succeeds. Over the next decade or so, it is highly likely that the criteria set out above for eligibility for Legal Aid may change and become ever more restrictive, in line with the general tightening of fiscal belts, as well as political pressures over the escalating costs of the UK Legal System.

If Legal Aid is a closed avenue, then other possibilities might include a legal expenses insurance claim, or approaching a trade union for support for a case contribution. If all else fails, then the claimant will have to bear the cost of the case preparations, such as the various expert reports and the time of the legal team. The best scenario would be that the pre-action protocols (see Section 2.6) are successful and the case is concluded to both parties' satisfaction prior to any court action. At worst, the solicitor will make the claimant aware that a demanding, expensive and glacially slow legal process will follow and a serious discussion is warranted on the toll these processes might take from the already compromised physical and mental condition of the individual and their reserves of determination. It is possible that the Law Firm might decide, after initiating the case and receiving initial reports and testimony relating to the case, that it could fund the rest of the proceedings through a no-win-no-fee basis, but this cannot be counted upon. At this point, many cases cannot proceed due to ill-health or lack of funds to progress the claim.

2.5 Claim progression and possible outcomes

Assuming the funding of the case is settled, after initial discussions, the solicitor may feel that the claimant has a good case and even better, he or she has ex-work colleagues who are willing to provide supportive statements on the claimant's work conditions. Then, they will ask the claimant for a very detailed statement on their workplace, employers and the precise day-to-day nature of their tasks. The claimant will be required to list to their best recollection, every chemical to which they might have been exposed and what protective measures, if any, the employer instituted. The claimant's view of the employer's attitude to Health and Safety will be sought and as much relevant information will be extracted from the claimant in their own words. A detailed picture can then be built up of the occupational world the claimant inhabited for perhaps many decades. The solicitor's task is then to use the information supplied by the claimant to assemble two key platforms of the case; these will be the establishment of, firstly, the claimant's current and future health status and, secondly, a detailed picture of causality. Hence, exposure to a substance or substances can be linked as strongly as possible with the claimant's injury and the degree of culpability of the employer, in terms of their attitude and work environment.

2.6 Pre-action protocols

Perhaps contrary to public perception, the legal system, its practitioners, as well as prospective claimants (formerly known as plaintiffs) and defendants are all actually under a strong obligation to try to settle a dispute without recourse to the courts. In such 'pre-action matters', a series of steps has been devised to provide every opportunity for successful mediation between the employer and the claimant. Such a pathway is summarised under 'pre-action protocols', which do not strictly demand specific steps to be taken; rather, they achieve resolution through provision of detailed guidance such as the Ministry of Justice's Civil Procedure Rules on Pre-Action Protocols for Disease and Illness Claims [8]. The Ministry states that these protocols are a *code of good practice*, although they do not have the force of law and remain guidelines. However, it should be borne in mind that refusal to cooperate with them can meet with sanctions if the case does reach court proceedings. The protocols also recognise that some claimants may well be seriously or even terminally ill, and expedition procedures are detailed, particularly with conditions such as mesothelioma linked to blue asbestos exposure.

The protocols guide the potential claimant on how to ask the potential defendant, as well as third parties such as hospitals or General Practitioners, to provide all the evidence necessary to support their case. There are time limits for either side to observe, and non-disclosure can be met with a court order, if necessary. The guidelines also impose reasonable standards of courtesy, such as if the claimant decides not to proceed, he must inform the potential defendant. Once sufficient information has been gathered, a letter of claim must be drafted by the solicitor involved and written to a set format. This will put the facts of the case together chronologically, accompanied by what are referred to as the *main allegations of fault* and any financial losses incurred by the claimant. The letter will also refer to all documents relevant to the case as well as insurance details pertaining to funding of the case. It is not compulsory at this stage to provide a medical report although it is probably useful to include. If it is included, then the defendant can also arrange for their own medical report to be made, and both parties will see each other's reports when they are submitted. The protocols also contain guidelines on whether it is necessary for both parties to appoint other experts, such as a scientist to assess causation or an expert to assess costs of care. If experts are to be appointed, the parties have the option to challenge the appointments within a set time. The defendant must acknowledge the letter of claim within 21 days and provide a formal response in 90 days. Once all the relevant information and reports pertaining to the case have been circulated and studied, the protocols suggest that suitable offers could be made by either side to resolve the issue. If the issue cannot be resolved in this fashion, or if the defendants decide to ignore the letter of claim, then the claimant may proceed to court action.

Due to the processes described earlier and for other reasons, the majority of cases will never reach a court. Cases might be settled out of court because the defendants suspect that they will incur less financial loss if they make a deal. Indeed, as in criminal law, both sides in a civil dispute will to some extent, metaphorically 'square up' to each other, like opposing armies in Napoleonic times. In criminal law, to force the court to go through a trial and be convicted usually means a fairly severe sentence for putting everyone to the trouble of the process. So it is not unusual that a guilty plea will be dramatically entered only at the very last minute, when it is clear to the defendant's legal team that all the appropriate witnesses have actually appeared, bearing damning testimony; indeed, the witnesses may well be standing nervously outside in the corridor next to the accused's family and several friends who were all present on that fateful night, but mysteriously are not part of the case. Similarly, in civil disputes, the side that assembles the most formidable case may well leave with a favourable settlement.

It is also apparent that even after the claim form has been issued and court action begins, many cases stall at different stages of the legal process, for a host of reasons. Even if the case is actually about to be heard in court, the claimant's solicitor will advise the claimant that legal proceedings are essentially unpredictable and an unfavourable outcome may occur despite the strength of the evidence and the logic and quality of the case preparation. If the case is settled privately, this may not be very satisfactory for an individual who feels a strong sense of injustice, although it is often the best deal they are likely to receive. Failure to accept what is perceived as a fair out-of-court settlement could lead to a very high cost bill, even if the claimant is successful. In addition, many claimants may well not be physically or mentally strong enough to face a remorseless verbal scything from a top-flight barrister.

2.7   Case initiation: Legal steps

Once pre-action issues are concluded and no agreement can be reached, the solicitor will continue with the case to accumulate all the relevant documents and reports, along with the claimant's statement and supportive statements from work colleagues. The claim is legally initiated by bringing it to the High or County Court. The claim is detailed in a Claim Form (formerly known as a 'writ'), and an accompanying 'Particulars of Claim', which is all intended to outline the main facts of the case, who is issuing proceedings against whom, why and how much they want as a remedy for the claim. This claim **must** contain a report from a medical practitioner concerning the injuries that are described within the claim. Once sealed by the Office in the Court, the claim is then regarded as 'issued' and then served on the defendants, who are now legally aware that a case is being prepared against them. Once duly served, the defendant must decide whether to fight the case or accept it. The defendant can then either counterclaim or lodge a defence which summarises their position. If the defence is obviously weak and/or the defendant fails to respond to the claim, then the claimant can receive judgement in their favour. If the defence appears robust, then the case will proceed. As in pre-action protocols, the two parties then provide the court with all the documentation related to the case, such as all the sworn witness statements and both parties can see each other's case.

At this point, the claimant can request that the defendant discloses all information which may be relevant to the case. This 'disclosure' (formerly known as 'discovery') is a particularly important stage, as with an occupational claim, large amounts of documents related to working practices, such as responses to worker's questions, information related to particular chemicals or their handling, may all have important bearing on the case. The defendant is legally obliged to disclose information, even that which is harmful to their own case, and there should not be any form of evidence tampering or destruction. If disclosure reveals that the Company knew of a particularly dangerous practice and a series of 'smoking gun' documents come to light, then the parties could well settle, as the case would clearly not be defensible in court. With an occupational case, disclosure may reveal a great deal of technically complex information which might require interpretation by expert testimony. In addition, medical examination material will also require explanation, and the claimant and the defence will then seek permission of the court to call more expert witnesses to support their respective cases. For more complete and detailed information on how civil cases are conducted, the reader is referred to the current version of the Queen's Bench Guide [9].

2.8 Expert reports: Medical

The pre-action process will have provided all the relevant medical records of the claimant and may well have led to the commissioning of an initial medical report or reports which should have accompanied the Letter of Claim. In the past, it was often deemed sufficient in a medical report to just detail the claimant's problems and injuries. However, for some time, it has been expected that the medical report 'substantiates' the claimant's injury, in the sense that attribution or causation must also be discussed which leaves the court in no doubt that other factors were unlikely to have caused the claimant's injury. This is important for the defence, who must be fully aware of the causation arguments which the claim will rely upon, so it can prepare an adequate response such as commissioning its own reports. The degree of credibility of this causation discussion in a medical report is naturally linked to the practitioner's experience in the area. Reports submitted in the past by some practitioners have been ruled partially or entirely inadmissible as evidence. Either the court did not consider that their methods of assessment of the claimant's medical condition were valid, or that the clinical judgements of the report were credible, or the practitioner could not show sufficient personal clinical or scientific credibility to support their causation and attribution assertions.

Consequently, for the purposes of a firm foundation for a case, a medical report will usually be the opinion of a senior consultant in the medical specialty relevant to the injury. This individual will have had experience of treating or examining claimants with similar occupationally linked diseases. They will review all the available medical records and examine the claimant. The consultant will then compile a report on the extent of their injury, as well as its impact on quality of life, future work prospects or, in severe cases, life expectancy. Alongside this report, the claimant's medical records will also be an important part of the case, and these will contain the claimant's entire medical history. This will comprise records of prior multiple consultations, treatment courses and outcomes, as well as detailed comment and opinion on the claimant's state of mental as well as physical health. This information is useful, as many different practitioners contribute their observations, so providing a fairly objective perspective on the claimant's health and behaviour. In addition, the claimant may often have been accompanied by their spouse in such consultations, and comment is often made on the influence of the spouse on the claimant's attitudes regarding their condition and who they believe to be responsible for it. In some cases, if the individual is deceased, then a pathologist or histologist may be called upon to provide a report on the condition of the individual, which may contribute to the Coroner's verdict, which in turn may have a strong bearing on any future claims related to the death. This could also involve examination of any tissue samples which might have been preserved, or even another post-mortem, in some cases.

If the claimant is still living, the medical evidence is usually reasonably straightforward, and the medical consultant or consultants should be able to authoritatively pronounce on the condition of the individual, as well as supply their perspective on causation. Many of us will have heard from relatives about the dreaded pronouncement made by a Hospital Consultant on life expectancy after a cancer diagnosis, and these predictions, apart from the occasionally fortunate individual, are usually fairly accurate. Hence, the medical report carries a great deal of weight, substance and sympathy to a case. At court, the doctor will be questioned on their experience with the condition and its links to occupation, and their recommendations will be viewed in the light of this experience. If the claimant is deceased and the cause of death is disputed, then the medical evidence will be as hotly contested as that of the scientific contributors to the case.

2.9 Causality: The scientific report

However, compelling and harrowing the medical condition of the claimant might be, this is not enough to make the case 'fly' and the onus is entirely on the claimant's legal team to convince the court on causation, which is sometimes termed 'attribution'. Causation is, of course, the link between the disease and the occupation. Legally, it could be viewed that a given condition is not actually an injury unless it can be directly linked to the accident or events that caused it. To a scientist, this could at face value appear to be simply a case of an explanation of perhaps how a chemical causes cancer at a cellular level. However, from the court's perspective, causation is much more detailed than this. Essentially, the court must see a clearly delineated progression of information which links a chemical with a condition, which is just as precise and sure as the linking of the murder weapon to the victim and perpetrator in a criminal trial. In the context of a murder trial, we are used to seeing on various television shows the process whereby DNA, gunshot residue and various other items inevitably chain the major players in the drama together. This process is complex, and just as in real-life murder trials, it is not always possible to link the participants with much more than circumstantial evidence and the barrister's art may be necessary to challenge and test the credibility of these links.

2.10 Recruiting the scientific expert

Of course, the links cannot be made without a high-quality scientific report, and the solicitor involved will approach a scientist with a background which is appropriate to the chemicals involved in the case. This approach will of course be based on the claimant's statement, where they detail all the agents to which they were exposed. The legal team might approach the scientist from a variety of standpoints, ranging from an online search, word of mouth or previous dealings, to approaches through university lists of experts in various fields. From the scientist's point of view, a solicitor may make an initial approach, involving a very brief outline of the case and information available to date.

The scientist will obviously then contact the solicitor to find out more about the case and make a judgement as to whether they feel that their expertise is appropriate to the case. The clearest and most direct credibility comes from published work in reputable journals over several years on the agent or agents in question, or closely related agents in the same class. An academic in a university might be required to teach in areas which are related to his subject area, but around which he or she does not necessarily have a publication record. Similarly, it is reasonable for a scientific expert to write a report on an area which is related fairly closely to his subject where he publishes, but there is always a danger of straying too far outside one's expertise. There is perhaps no hard and fast rule about this, but it must be decided mostly by the scientist themselves. One must feel comfortable in interpreting and explaining information in the required area, and if necessary, it helps to imagine being cross-examined by a barrister in a court. However, the final measure must be whether a prospective expert report writer feels that he or she would prosper if they were cross-examined by an expert who had published extensively in that field. This is probably the toughest test of credibility in terms of minutely detailed knowledge. It is little wonder that it is not easy for solicitors to find individuals who have the necessary knowledge of a subject area, let alone the confidence to argue over fine points of science in a court.

2.11   Expectations of the expert: The court

In the past, expert evidence was, in some cases, treated with a credibility that it did not deserve and some infamous cases are on record, where individuals were convicted on the evidence of an 'expert' who had built their career on the identification of a particular psychological condition, and it was clearly in that expert's interest and credibility that this condition was to be identified in several defendants, whose lives were ruined in the ensuing proceedings. In other cases, some experts would act as 'guns for hire' and say in court what they thought would support the case of the party that was paying them. In yet other circumstances, medical and scientific expert reports have been ruled inadmissible as evidence, as either the expert was not qualified in the eyes of the court or that the reports departed from objectivity to the point that they looked suspiciously like 'crusades' on behalf of their clients. The role of the expert is now much more clearly defined in Civil Proceedings, and this is part of the process which is intended to reach a just and fair settlement, through encouraging consensus in what remains an adversarial process.

It is important to see that the expert currently can take on one of two major roles in the preparation of a case. A legal team responsible for mounting a claim can appoint an expert **advisor** who is not likely to give evidence in the case, but is present to guide either party in their work with the case. This individual is under obligation to give both sides of any potential argument and should discuss frankly the strengths and weaknesses of both sides' positions. Either side could appoint an expert advisor, and his or her instructions are likely to be 'privileged', that is, not disclosable to the opposition. This is partly because, at this stage, arguments are still being formulated and the case is still in the process of preparation. In other situations, this expert could be appointed as an expert advisor to the court, and in that case, he will be issued with new instructions (his old instructions will remain privileged) which are open to all to read and his duty then is to the court, rather than to the original party that hired him.

The second role an expert can take on is the more 'traditional' expert **witness**. In this capacity, the expert acts essentially as a court appointed independent and impartial witness. Indeed, it is required that at the end of their written report, they write a declaration from the Queen's Bench Guide [9]:

> 7.9.2 The duty of an expert called to give evidence is to assist the court. This duty overrides any obligation to the party instructing him or by whom s/he is being paid (see the Part 35 Practice Direction). In fulfilment of this duty, an expert must for instance make it clear if a particular question or issue falls outside his/her expertise or if he or she considers that insufficient information is available on which to express an opinion.

Hence, the expert may well be paid by the claimant, but he is not 'owned' by the claimant's legal team and cannot, for example, under any circumstances supply a favourable opinion for the claimant because he or she feels very sympathetic to the claimant's predicament. In effect, the court will decide how many experts are allowed to participate in a case, and indeed, the court may either allow both parties to instruct different experts or even dictate that both parties actually instruct the same expert. This latter course is most likely to occur if the court needs the expert to inform it on facts rather than opinion. However, other cases may hinge on expert opinion, so then the claimant and the defendant will organise their own experts.

If experts are in the same discipline or field, the court will most likely order them to confer, either by meeting or by some other means. This can allow the court to determine what is agreed between the opposing parties and what is not. If the experts change their position as a result of the meeting, then this has to be conveyed to the respective parties and, if necessary, the court itself.

The expert's written report must contain the instructions they have been given by either or both parties in the claim. Once the parties in the case have settled on their choice of experts, it is strongly discouraged for them to abandon an expert and use another, in pursuit of a more favourable impact on their case. If an expert's services are no longer sought by either party, their original report will remain part of the evidence of the case. It is also important to realise, as an expert witness, that after submission of your report, the other party can write to the expert requesting clarification of specific points within reason, and this may occur up to 28 days after the report is submitted, although in some cases it can occur further down the line if the court allows it. Questions to experts are strictly regulated by the court to prevent excessive numbers of queries. Section 7.9 of the current Queen's Bench Guide [9] is necessary reading for experts in terms of how their contribution is managed by the court. Ultimately, a case might hinge on the strength of the causality report from an expert, so it is interesting to consider how a solicitor might view a prospective expert and how the expert themselves reacts to the unfamiliar legal process.

2.12   Expectations of the expert: The solicitor/ expert relationship

Regarding the contrasting attitudes of the legal team and the expert, both will naturally be acutely aware that they inhabit different professional spheres; the solicitor may be concerned about how well the expert's report supports the case and also how robust the expert may be in the witness stand. The naive expert may also be concerned as to how their possible report might be evaluated or assessed and, if it came to court, how would they respond to the classic worst-case legal verbal savaging. At this point, it is probably worthwhile examining some parallels between legal examination of evidence and the medico-scientific process of data handling and publication. Just as most scientists and doctors are not necessarily aware of the legal process, solicitors are usually unlikely to be aware of how experts publish their work. As part of their normal duties, laboratory scientists and some clinically qualified scientists write manuscripts for publication, where they carefully compile their findings into relatively digestible tracts which are meticulously worded descriptions of what they did, how and why it was done and what the findings actually mean in the context of the field. These manuscripts are then submitted to journals which send them out for peer review, usually to the authors' competitors, who may or may not be their sworn enemies in their field. These reviewers often spend a disproportionate amount of their time subjecting the manuscripts to a forensic dismantling which usually exposes the various flaws in the approach, methods or interpretations. The reviewers will then write a comprehensive report (containing more than a few painstakingly crafted barbs), which the editor will use to decide whether publication of the findings is worthwhile.

Whilst one's scientific arch nemesis (isn't an ordinary nemesis enough?) may reach for his metaphorical sharpened stake, mallet and garlic to try to obliterate the manuscript under the cloak of anonymity, if the work is basically well executed, is novel and advances science, then it is likely it will survive the intellectual kicking it will receive. In practice, the editor could reject the work as unworthy or beyond repair, or he or she might invite the authors to refute the coruscating review step by step, in a process which can take the authors' days and sometimes weeks. This involves the painstaking dissection of the reviewer's points and the drafting of appropriate responses and, if required, carrying out more experiments (groan), as well as changes to the structure and content of the manuscript. This is intellectually and physically exhausting, but, essential to the progression of science and medicine and under the auspices of a decisive, yet fair editor and a good journal, will lead to a much improved manuscript. Therefore, it is important that solicitors are aware that laboratory and clinical scientists are well versed in defending their work from literally everything their enemies can hurl at them. Indeed, scientists' careers depend on the ability to use patient and complex written arguments to methodically refute the reviewer's contentions, using published evidence to support their case. Equally, scientific and medical experts should be aware that in the preparation of a causality report for a solicitor, a very similar review process will occur initially at the level of those that are preparing and participating in the mounting of the case, such as the claimant's legal team, as well as that of the opposition. Hence, it is vital that the expert enters the process of drafting a causality report with the same level of dedication that is required to publish a manuscript in a high-quality journal in their field. Indeed, the expert should be prepared for some very direct and sometimes painful criticism of their report's ideas, structure, approach and detail.

Laboratory scientists in particular, are often perceived as existing in their proverbial ivory tower, sealed off from society in a rarefied existence of intellectual discourse with their peers. Whilst this is not always the case, it is perhaps conceivable that some highly accomplished scientists might feel that they are unlikely to meet their intellectual superior outside of their field. However, in dealing with counsel, experts in general should take into account that legal training and practice requires a formidable combination of vast memory for detail, exceptional plasticity of mind to master briefs and situations, as well as velocity of incisive intellectual analysis that laboratory scientists are not often required to display. Indeed, many of us dwell perhaps a tad too comfortably in our familiar fields deploying our usual well-honed and, dare I say it, complacent arguments. This attitude has been noted in other experts; in 1989, Mikhail Timofeyevich Kalashnikov (1919-2013) witheringly described his fellow designers' devotion to their ideas, as 'like a spinster to her cats'. In dealing with lawyers, therefore, all experts should be prepared to be extremely attentive and flexible if necessary when they meet to discuss reports and other aspects of a case.

Whilst a solicitor might be convinced that an expert could mount a detailed argument in a written report, he or she might be less confident that an expert could defend their position in court under cross-examination by a barrister and perhaps when faced with contradictory reports from the experts from the opposing team. Equally, an expert who has not submitted a report of this type before and has not given evidence in court might also feel certain trepidation in facing such a perceived ordeal. It is, however, important to consider that laboratory and clinical scientists do receive training in this area in scientific meetings when presenting their work. Many scientists and clinicians, as well as their Ph.D. students are exposed to aggressive and incisive questioning in public (which might appear to the bystander as a mauling) from their competitors that requires a series of rapid yet convincing reposts. Indeed, performances at meeting question periods can have a crucial bearing on a scientist's future career. Hence, it is useful for both scientists and solicitors to consider that scientists are actually surprisingly well prepared for their day in court. It is also worth mentioning that even if clinician experts have not participated in scientific and medical meetings, they will have been subjected to ruthless criticism from their peers as they ascend their career ladder, so they too are more than capable of holding their own when giving evidence.

2.13   The expert report: The contract

After the expert agrees to supply the report, it is important to realise that rather like the pet that is more than just for Christmas, once the expert agrees to participate, they are inextricably bound to the case until it is concluded. If their report is submitted as part of the evidence in legal proceedings, then the expert may be called to give evidence and can be legally compelled to do so under pain of serious legal sanction. Usually, the solicitor will ask the expert for some estimate of the 'reasonable' costs involved in the preparation of the report. The expert should cost their report by using a realistic system which reflects the true cost of their time and access to appropriate resources. Most universities have no objection to academics acting as consultants to various organisations, as it adds to prestige, and the academic to an extent 'trades' on the reputation of their university as much as their own research credibility. Indeed, the position of the expert, either as academic, clinician, or commercial scientist, adds to their independence from the process of the case. Therefore, a realistic estimate of the costs in terms of the time that the expert will put into the case should be tabled. If the work is to be carried out in the expert's free time, then the individual can, to some extent, charge what they believe the market will stand. If the expert will be writing the report in work time, then this must also be allowed for in the final calculation. For instance, with the prior agreement of the University, a fee could be directed to a fund which could be used to support laboratory work, for example, or could be taken as personal income.

In estimating the cost, just as an individual might object strongly if a tradesman suddenly revised his estimate of a fee violently upwards, the expert must stick to their initial estimate of the cost of the report and stipulate whether this will include or exclude revisions to the report. It is often difficult to estimate how long it might take to compile a report, but it is important not to under- or over-cost it. The ability to cost a report accurately usually improves dramatically with experience.

Regarding arrangements for report delivery, then the solicitor may require the report by a specific date with respect to oncoming court proceedings, so the expert must agree to supply the report with respect to the timeframe required. With respect to payment, as the expert is the one sought in this situation, this is the only occasion when he or she has control of the relationship, in terms of the power to dictate the conditions of payment before they agree to supply the report. It is also worth mentioning that once the legal team are in receipt of your report, there can be little incentive for them to attend to your remuneration in an expeditious manner. Therefore, the optimal terms should be something akin to the expert agreeing a date to produce the report and then a few days beforehand, they should notify the solicitor that the report is ready. The solicitor will have secured the payment from the claimant and then the money is passed on to the expert or their University and the report is then handed over on receipt of the payment. If the solicitor does not agree to these payment terms, then the standard response should be something polite, such as 'by all means please feel free to seek the services of another expert'. As with online auctions, when the money appears, the report will be sent.

2.14 Compiling the report

Over the past decade, the requirements of an expert report have been improved dramatically, and the report must fulfil several objectives. Firstly, it must establish quickly the credibility of the expert. Secondly, it must include the material instructions to the expert, thirdly, it should trace causality and, fourthly, it must be supplied to assist the court as detailed earlier and therefore cannot be 'partisan'. Credibility is established with a paragraph of the expert's qualifications and experience, which eventually focusses on the area of expertise involved and might include numbers of publications in the area. Other information, such as courses taught and books contributed to or even written, would all be beneficial in convincing the court that you have the credibility required to participate in the case. Then, it is necessary to state the 'mission' so to speak, such as instructions received from the solicitor with regard to determination of causation. The expert should read all the disclosure documentation, medical reports, medical records, as well as claimant and employer witness statements available carefully and note down the main points related to the case. This can amount to suitcases full of documents which must be examined, and this reading period is rather difficult to cost into the estimate of the fee. It might be worthwhile asking the solicitor handling the case approximately how much there is in terms of the physical quantity of disclosure material and what form it takes. The solicitor should provide at least a rough estimate of this, although one I received was summarised in the phrase … 'wheelbarrowloads, mate', which was reasonably accurate.

2.15 The toxin or toxins

Perhaps the first area to approach should be a contextual description of the nature of the possible toxin, followed by some description of its uses and its mode of toxicity. In some cases, a specific chemical agent might have been identified by the claimant, or by the defendant, or both, and it is beyond question what the agent actually is. With such a single chemical, then it is relatively straightforward to describe its place in any given industrial process and the course of exposure and subsequent causation can be mapped reasonably easily. However, at the other extreme, a claimant might have been exposed to a considerable variety of different substances for different time periods and even in different environments for a number of employers over their working lives. In this case, it is unlikely that the claimant really can remember which agent may have caused his problems and indeed, he may only have the most vague and tentative identification of the various chemicals that he encountered. This is particularly prevalent in claims relating to agrochemicals, as well as in engineering and the writer must use whatever sketchy information is available in the claimant's statement to piece together the actual chemicals involved.

   The claimant's statement might refer to agents used up to 40 years previously, and in some cases, the description can be as vague as 'it came in a big blue drum', which does not appear to be terribly helpful. However, even in such a case, a colleague might remember what was written on the drum, and the substance can be identified through a memory of part or whole of a trade name; such is the power of the internet that the chemical can then usually be traced. It is then sometimes found that a trade name could still be used, but the mix of chemicals used in that preparation in 1968, for example, has changed markedly and bears little or no resemblance to its most recent incarnation, despite the agent remaining available from the same manufacturer and that it even performs the same function. In one report I compiled, the big blue drum was recalled by a colleague of a claimant to have 'Genk' printed on the side. This could easily be identified as 'Genklene', which was 1,1,1-trichloroethane, a chlorinated solvent manufactured by ICI from 1960 which was used as a degreaser in a range of industries, from electronics manufacture to automotive and light engineering processes until legislation in the United States, and the European Union in the 1990s began to restrict usage of ozone-depleting chlorohydrocarbons [10, 11]. This meant that alternatives had to be found to agents such as 1,1,1-trichloroethane.

However, degreasing remains an integral part of metal preparation in manufacturing. Hence, various new processes, based on water/detergent mixes, alcohols, ketones and non-chlorinated solvents had to be created to replace this solvent. Manufacturing processes therefore do evolve to attempt to reduce hazards, but not always successfully (see Chapter 6, section 7.1).

Regarding the claimant exposed to multiple agents, in such cases, it can be that some of the substances are just not relevant to the case as they are not particularly toxic or dangerous. The writer must painstakingly research each agent to establish this and hopefully narrow down the potentially toxic agents which he or she believes might be the causative toxins relating to the claimant's current condition. At this point in the report, the writer will have read a great deal of detail on the nature of the chemicals and their specific toxic effects. It is very useful at this stage when reading the claimant's statement and the disclosure to search carefully for 'signature' symptoms reported by the claimant during his daily working life, or data or descriptions from medical reports which can be linked with prior exposure to a particular toxin or chemical. Whilst not exactly the 'smoking gun', such effects support the case that the agent entered the claimant in sufficient quantity to cause significant acute symptoms; for example, solvents are known to cause effects on behaviour, although many factors influence behaviour, not just solvents. It would be preferable to find some clear evidence that the claimant really had been exposed to the agent. In cases of exposure to the solvent dichloromethane, this agent is metabolised to carbon monoxide, which could be measured as carboxyhaemoglobin in a hospital CO-Oximeter. If such evidence shows high CO exposure, then assuming other CO sources can be discounted, this suggests that the solvent entered the claimant in considerable quantity at least on the occasion of measurement. This can in turn be used to support other contentions on the solvent's effect on behaviour.

Likewise, we are all aware that alcoholic drinks consumed in high quantity can cause nausea and vomiting. Exposure to organophosphate insecticides interferes with liver enzyme function, causing the consumption of only small amounts of alcohol to result in nausea and vomiting. In a claimant who is a regular drinker, who is suddenly violently sick after only a single alcoholic drink, this suggests a considerable and very recent exposure to an organophosphate, providing all other causes of such acute sickness can be ruled out. All these observations outline the daily series of acute exposures which taken together form chronic exposure, which can then be linked with the claimant's current problems.

2.16   Toxin entry

Whether the claimant was exposed to a variety of agents which were known or unknown and before causality can be established, the key first stage is demonstrating how the chemical entered the claimant's body. If a chemical causes a strong pharmacological effect as detailed in the previous section, then it is self-evident that it has entered the body in some quantity, and local tissue toxicity effects may well highlight the route of entry. If a claim is linked to a more subtle effect, such as carcinogenicity, then there may be some doubt as to how the agent entered the body, so careful consideration must be made to establishing routes of entry.

From first principles, the toxin or toxins could only enter by mouth, through inspired air, or somehow pass through the skin. The report must address this issue in detail and provide a convincing account of how the claimant might have received their daily 'dosage' of the chemical. It is useful to consider these three points of entry. It is unlikely that most workers would ingest a chemical, unless they had handled it without gloves and then consumed food and drink with contaminated hands. Similarly, it would be regarded as irresponsible to deliberately contaminate oneself without regard to the consequences or engaged in patently unsafe work practices, such as the habit of some car mechanics in Nigeria, where they used to spray mouthfuls of petrol at car parts to clean them. So the most likely routes of entry into the claimant will be inhalation and/or absorption through the skin. This latter organ is the body's largest and is a highly effective barrier to most substances, particularly water-based agents. The skin has evolved to keep our water content in and external water out and can be relied upon to provide an effective barrier to many toxins. Even cyanide, for all its potential lethality, cannot enter the body through skin; it must be ingested. However, the skin can be vulnerable to some oil-based agents and can present little if any barrier effect towards some solvents, which can disrupt its structure and penetrate it. In addition, such solvents can also 'carry' other toxic agents in solution across the skin into the blood. Perhaps the best example of the surprising vulnerability of the skin is the solvent dimethyl sulphoxide (DMSO). Many life scientists will attest to inadvertently touching a splash of DMSO on a lab surface and within less than 10 min, a vile taste enters the mouth. The DMSO would have entered the skin, passed straight through to the blood, then to the liver, where it is metabolised to sulphides, which then reach the salivary glands and saliva to be tasted.

Another important feature of the skin is that it is not uniform in thickness and vulnerability. Skin on the feet or the hands is obviously thicker than perhaps skin on the torso, for example, and might be more resistant to toxin penetration. As outlined with the unfortunate mule spinners in Chapter 1, scrotal skin is vastly more permeable to solvents, compared with the skin on the hands, and clearly a chemical may only have a short distance to travel before it encounters the testes, and it will gain access to their blood supply, which is the gateway to the rest of the body. As we will see from the reports in the next chapters, workers often wear highly contaminated clothing on a daily basis, which offers little or no protection against oily toxic substances.

The lung is quite different to the skin in that it has evolved to be the very reverse of a barrier – it is intended to absorb gases from the atmosphere and convey them to the blood extremely efficiently. All smokers will attest to the time period of perhaps 15 s or so, when the nicotine from the first cigarette of the day satisfies their craving. Hence, the lung is extremely vulnerable to a variety of gaseous products, such as different solvents, as well as 'aerosols'. These can range from what most people would regard as 'smoke' through to quite dense air suspensions of particles, which can contain a range of substances, from metals to fluids. Whilst solvents are absorbed rapidly and very efficiently, particulate matter is resisted more effectively by the lung, through the actions of hair-like projections on the bronchial tree known as cilia. These trap large (larger than 50 μm) particles in mucous and waft them upwards towards the throat where they can be coughed out, or swallowed, reaching the stomach and the gastrointestinal tract, to be eliminated in faeces. Particles in the sub-10-μm category will reach the alveoli, the tiny air–blood interface sacs which are the most basic unit of the lung's function. From this point, the particles could be engulfed by immune system cells, and if this process triggers an inflammatory response, then the lungs can be damaged directly by a toxin, as well as indirectly by the process of the immune response.

2.17 Toxin chemical nature

Whilst the nature of the tissues which encounter the toxin is important in how the agent enters the claimant, the physicochemical properties of the chemical or substance are also vital in relation to how easily or rapidly this process occurs. If the chemical involved is very water soluble, but has a high molecular weight, then it will not pass through skin, and relatively basic protective clothing will be an adequate barrier, so exposure would be more likely to occur through inhalation, but this would perhaps depend on the presence of a very heavy aerosol which would in turn require quite high working temperatures to maintain its presence. If an agent was of lower molecular weight, it might exist in a vapour/aerosol form which could be easily breathed if working temperatures were lower. Either way, the water solubility of the agent would restrict its entry to the claimant to inhalation.

In contrast, very oil-soluble agents might enter through skin as well as through inhalation. A combination of an oil-soluble agent and volatile solvents present on surfaces, or thrown from rotating surfaces, such as that seen in the cotton industry in the early twentieth century, would ensure entry of the oils through inhalation and through the skin. If the agent has a high molecular weight, this might restrict its entry, but other solvents could effectively 'carry' it into the claimant. Perhaps the most dangerous combination of these factors would be low molecular weight, volatility and oil solubility, such as is seen in organic solvents, which often have specific toxic effects once they enter the body. Such exposures are well recognised in the workplace in most developed countries, to the point where many processes which create dense mists of such solvents are now either fully automated or the worker wears a complete protective suit and has a separate air supply, as in automotive paint spraying. In the expert report to this point, the scientific literature will provide detailed information on the physicochemical nature of the agent and its likely routes of entry and journal or book articles can be referenced to provide a clear path of credibility through the report.

2.18   Exacerbating factors in toxin absorption

After establishing the nature of the agent and its likely points of entry into the claimant's body, it is important to evaluate their working environment's contribution to accentuating or minimising these factors. Obviously, the information needed to illuminate this area of the report is gleaned from the claimant's, as well as his colleagues' respective statements, plus information from the defendant revealed in the disclosure, which might contradict that of the claimant. The claimant's statement will provide details of work processes and their degree of day-to-day protection from the processes, with respect to standard operating procedures related to health and safety, protective clothing, design and type of machinery, absence or presence of guards on the machinery, the degree of cleanliness of the working environment (ambient air and surfaces) and all other information pertaining to the progression of the chemical from drum or vessel to the claimant's body. Whilst much of this information might conflict, it is up to the writer to try to find a common thread through the various accounts of what the defendant believed were the working conditions and what the claimant reported. As we have seen in Chapter 1, many industrial environments in the distant and even relatively recent past were extremely hostile, regarding noise, air pollution and sustained high temperatures. If most of the accounts point to a hot and heavily polluted, poorly maintained and unpleasant environment, then high temperatures and lack of air extraction would promote the existence of oily toxic 'fogs' which would add to physical contamination caused by shortcomings in protective clothing. Other factors, such as shift patterns and restrictions of toilet breaks, all conspire to increase the presence of the toxin in the working environment and actively hinder its removal from the body through excretion of urine. Indeed, conditions of high humidity and reduced fluid intake would increase the toxicity of agents which are unstable in urine, such as aromatic amine metabolites, which target the urinary bladder in their carcinogenicity, as discussed in Chapter 4. The report must present a realistic picture of the degree of daily 'dosage' or systemic exposure the claimant endured during his working life.

2.19   Causation: Mechanisms

Once the case has been made that a working environment does promote the entry of a potential toxin to the claimant, the next step is to use the scientific literature again to describe how the compound actually injured the claimant and led to their current state. A solicitor might outline to the expert in their instructions that the claimant has to show that there is a reasonable probability that the toxin caused the injuries described. This 'reasonable probability' has been described as a much lower probability than scientific proof. For example, one solicitor outlined to me the difference between these two standards of proof as being '51 compared with 98%'. So the question is being asked of the expert whether it is biologically plausible for the health issues to be caused by the toxin. However, whether the expert can make a case for biological plausibility does to a large extent depend on scientific, medical and legal precedents.

In the case of known toxins, such as aromatic amines and bladder cancer, there is a very strong scientific and medical literature which establishes precedent on these agents in several industries, such as the automotive, tyre, printing and dye industries. In legal processes, we often read about 'test cases' where precedent might be set in a particular area. In the legal evaluation of occupational toxicity, the court will look in a report for a strong scientific precedent to support a case. So if a claimant has bladder cancer and it is possible to prove that they were exposed to an agent such as β-naphthylamine (BNA), then there are plenty of publications to cite which illustrate the link. However, even in this area, with a large literature on bladder cancer and carcinogenesis, this is not straightforward. As mentioned earlier, the most potent *known* bladder carcinogens such as BNA have long been removed from the workplace, so the process of finding scientific support for other specific human bladder carcinogens is surprisingly difficult. Indeed, there are plenty of agents which are proven carcinogens in animals, but it can be more difficult to show that a chemical is demonstrably carcinogenic in humans. This means that if the claimant has a condition which is associated with occupation and the 'usual chemical suspects' are not immediately detectable, to the scientist, this would seem straightforward. He or she would search for papers and reports which implicated other agents in high incidences of bladder cancer. To the court, however, such an approach might not be enough to prove that the occupational experience was causative, as a specific agent cannot be identified. Indeed, in bladder cancer, there is a scientific literature linking polycyclic aromatic hydrocarbons to the condition, but this is a weaker association with the cancer compared with that of aromatic amines, although there are signs that this situation may change as more data is published (see Chapter 4, section 12).

In other cases, a chemical might be well established to be acutely toxic, but not necessarily linked convincingly with chronic toxicity. Or there may be a literature linking a particular agent with a condition, which is not accepted as a proven case by the scientific and medical establishment. Either way, the report writer must assemble a case which contains a balanced appraisal of all shades of opinion, and although the writer may feel the agent might be causative, other experts could contest this extremely strongly. Clearly, for the credibility of the report writer, if other experts do disagree, they should not be able to cite important literature that the original report writer has omitted as he or she felt that those reports did not support their case. So it is essential that all the important and relevant literature is cited.

In explaining causation, it is imperative that the descriptions should be accurate, but not festooned in jargon. It is worth echoing the sentiments described earlier that legal minds are sharp and should not be underestimated, and clearly explained anatomical, biochemical and physiological processes can be rendered understandable to the intelligent layman. If necessary, analogies can be made if they are sufficiently accurate and well drafted to explain a point rapidly and precisely. As mentioned previously, the report should read in the same way as a scientific journal, with perhaps a few concessions to the lay reader such as avoidance of too many acronyms and abbreviations.

2.20 Contemporaneous knowledge

How much *did* an organisation know of the dangers of particular chemicals or processes at the time they were being used, and how much *should* they have known about these dangers? This is a crucial issue in a report, which can be very difficult to assess and somewhat subjective. For example, It would appear at first glance to be fair comment that the dangers of smoking were not generally known to the industry or the general public perhaps as late as the 1950s and 1960s as successive Hollywood stars and sporting legends lined up to promote cigarettes. However, as far back as the early 1860s, it was common knowledge in Imperial Russia that cigarettes were dangerous, as they are directly referred to as such in Dostoyevsky's 'Crime and Punishment'. If we go further back, then for all his faults, such as his unhealthy obsession with witches and shockingly poor personal hygiene, James I (1567–1625), had a clear, prescient and characteristically bilious attitude to smoking in his tome *A Counterblaste to Tobacco* written in 1604. Reading his words, one wonders what an excellent and entertaining television critic he might have made. At the other extreme, for tobacco manufacturers to claim that they were unaware of the toxicity of their product as late as the 1980s was at the time, and is now, farcical. The question remains, when was it reasonable to assume that the average person would accept that they had a 50% chance of dying from a 40-year, 20-a-day cigarette habit.

The major medical epidemiological work condemning tobacco took place both before and immediately after World War II, although this conflict certainly set back the anti-smoking cause. While he waited to enter the Royal Navy, my 19-year-old father was sent to collect unexploded incendiary bombs with a bucket of sand and a spade during the 1941 Liverpool Blitz, and a bomb exploded in his face, temporarily blinding him. While he lay on a stretcher, as an act of kindness, somebody commenced his 31-year smoking habit by jamming a lighted unfiltered cigarette in his mouth. Although millions of persistent tobacco habits started under the extreme pressures of war, several influential publications appeared in the early 1950s highlighting the dangers of the substance. Certainly, Sir Richard Doll's landmark paper, which highlighted the impact of smoking on the medical profession itself [12] persuaded many doctors to stop smoking. Whilst epidemiological studies showing the health impact of tobacco were publicised to some extent and did eventually reach the popular press, unfortunately, the dangers of tobacco were not effectively conveyed to the public until decades later. Hence, it could be said that if it is this difficult to disseminate successfully such a vital health message to the public which had so much solid and reliable research behind it, it is little wonder that many toxic agents have remained in use in industry for far longer than they should have.

Today, when a study is published in the scientific press condemning a food, drug or product, the route through to the tabloid newspapers and the internet is almost instant. However, the reaction evoked is often mixed, as usually many published studies over several years are required to convince the scientific and medical professions over a particular issue, let alone the public. Indeed, the advice given to pregnant mothers on what constitutes 'safe' alcohol consumption is a good example of the lack of consistency of scientific advice over many years.

In Chapter 1, the tragic story of the mule spinners and their cancers led to major changes in the cotton industry, although the danger from the oils used did not appear to reach the motor industry for many years as we shall see in Chapter 4. Whilst aromatic hydrocarbons were known to be dangerous for perhaps half a century before their mechanisms of toxicity were uncovered, they remained in use in many other industries which were not aware of the problem, or worse, were aware, yet ignored it. The UK rubber industry eliminated BNA from the end of the 1940s, although many other tyre manufacturers around the world studiously ignored the danger until the 1970s. It could be viewed that once the dangers of a particular process or chemical, or a combination of process and chemical have been highlighted in several scientific or medical reports in good-quality journals and this information has filtered through to the specialist press of that industry, then even if the issue had not generally reached the public, then it is fair to say that the employers should have addressed the issue. In some instances, in disclosure documents, the process of an employer coming to terms with a potentially problematic and expensive issue relating to occupational health can be both illuminating and frustrating, as the issue is raised, explored, digested and then, in some cases, quietly allowed to slip away.

Clearly, there are degrees of culpability which will vary case by case. For instance, an employer may ignore an issue highlighted by other employers in the same industry, and the disclosure and contemporary publications make this apparent. In other cases, the employer might recognise the danger but, for whatever reason, fail to institute the necessary measures to protect the workforce. Again, the problem might have been flagged up and dealt with in terms of worker protection, but the protective technology was simply inadequate and the agent succeeded in causing injury to the workforce. Either way, it is necessary in the report to ensure that in so far as is possible, the writer must make some argument based on documentation and what could be reasonably known at the time, whether the employer did make adequate recognition and provision against the threat.

After the final statement to the effect that the expert's duty is to the court rather than whoever is paying for the report, a comprehensive reference list should be supplied with all the necessary citations checked to the standard expected in a journal submission.

2.21 The initial draft

Once the report is written and submitted, the legal team will consider it carefully in the light of all the available evidence of the case. Sometimes, developments can arise where more information becomes available or another relevant report appears. In this case, the report may require alteration or partial re-drafting to accommodate these developments. The solicitor handling the case will examine all the reports in detail to ensure that there are no inconsistencies, such as where one expert has referred to one issue and the other may have omitted it, or if there is confusion over the facts of the case. However, the court system strongly discourages attempts by legal teams to surreptitiously write an expert's report or significantly alter it in the absence of new information, again to augment their case. This is a slightly more complex area, as it is entirely reasonable for the legal team to peruse the draft carefully to consider its impact, and with an inexperienced expert, it is fair to say that legal team could perhaps point out obvious 'hostages to fortune', which would not appear in a report from an expert well versed in legal report writing. There can also be instances where an expert has not included or considered a vital piece of evidence or publication, and such an omission does strongly impact the credibility and value of the report. It is also possible that parts of the report simply are too opaque for the legal team to understand. So in such cases, some revision is necessary; indeed, the legal team will ask for the report to be re-drafted to make it 'judge friendly'. This might involve some basic modifications to allow the judge to assimilate the information more quickly and also will facilitate making detailed and repeated references to specific areas of the report. It is now strongly recommended to break reports into short numbered paragraphs to make this process easier for the court to deal with.

2.22 Silence in court

The object of the expert's report is shared by the court, in so far as the report should provide a scientifically based assessment of how the toxic agent entered the claimant and inflicted the damage to his or her health. In addition, the expert's opinion on the culpability of the employer will also assist the court in arriving at a fair judgement. In many cases, the report alone will suffice and the expert will not be required to appear in court. However, an expert might be called to give evidence if the court requires it; there could be a dispute between experts, or the defendant's team might wish to explore different aspects of the case. Depending on the proceedings, the expert might have to give evidence in front of a judge, magistrates or a coroner. He or she might be questioned by the defendant's counsel and/or the magistrates, the coroner, or the judge. Until recently, all court proceedings were noted down by court stenographers, who were highly skilled individuals who used a special keyboard to note down the proceedings at the normal speed of human speech, which is about 180 words per minute. This is nearly twice as fast as a shorthand typist could manage, although occasionally individuals used to be asked to speak perhaps a little slower than usual to ensure the stenographer did not miss any of their testimony. However, a new system, known as Digital Audio Recording Transcription and Storage (Darts) has now largely replaced the stenographers, and the system was rolled out in March 2012.

Giving evidence in open court can be daunting, and it is stressful for the expert, as unless they have a parallel existence as a notably unsuccessful criminal, the environment and procedures are unfamiliar and the process feels very 'remotely managed'. It is not always predictable exactly when the expert might be called to give evidence, if they are indeed called at all.

The tone and style of questioning will, of course, be related to the questioner. A judge, coroner or magistrate will ask direct questions in measured tones mainly to gain some clarity concerning specific issues in order to master a complex case. This is clearly different from a barrister's line of questions which may be linked with clarity, or possibly may also be intended to discredit or undermine the witness's credibility and composure. Of course, we know that a barrister is tasked with winning a case by whatever fair means at his or her disposal. Whilst we have all watched fictional barristers in court, in real life, the most skilled barristers are every bit as capable, fluent, persuasive and ruthless as their TV equivalents. As an observer, it seems to me that rather than simply conduct a case, they inhabit it, like actors who immerse themselves in a role. The public often scorn highly paid individuals such as various lawyers and perhaps footballers, as they are seen as motivated entirely by money. However, it is clear that in many instances, the sheer intensity of a footballer's commitment is obviously visible at a game, and it indicates that there is no thought of money in their mind at that point. Indeed, as they say in the United States, winning isn't everything; it is the only thing. So barristers 'live' a case and might even simmer with indignation about the opposition's tactics in the court canteen over a somewhat dubious looking *moussaka*.

Hence, for the expert who is required to attend court as a witness and will be cross-examined, it is worthwhile considering that one way to be comprehensively and traumatically eviscerated by a barrister is to be unprepared or not fully aware of all the available information in a case. Whilst the court will treat an expert with appropriate respect, barristers can sometimes be determined to undermine an expert's credibility by any means that come to hand. It is also worth remembering that judges are well known to vary as to how much latitude they may allow a barrister as he or she develops their line of questioning. Clearly, in this environment, the expert needs to be ready to stand their ground and look after themselves. So prior to a court appearance, it is important to re-read the original report and all other documents relevant to the case to ensure that you are as prepared as you possibly can be to answer questions relevant to your claimed expertise.

This may all sound daunting, but a court appearance is probably not as difficult as perhaps a Ph.D. viva might have been. Other experiences are also relevant to a court appearance, such as job interviews, question sessions after presentations at scientific or medical meetings and events linked to subject area external teaching accreditations, where panels of experts might question individuals on specific topics for some period of time, for high stakes. Overall, an expert scientist or medical practitioner should feel confident that providing they have prepared thoroughly, they already possess the necessary skills and determination to comprehend barrister's arguments and avoid being led into difficult positions.

2.23   Report writing in the real world

Scientists and medical personnel will approach causation/medical assessment report writing from a variety of experiences. A medically trained individual may have worked extensively with clinical trials of one sort or another, or in the case of a pharmacist, with practice-related studies. Both approaches will involve patients and/or volunteers. A laboratory scientist may have had experience in clinical trial studies, either through trial planning and organisation, analysis of the samples or other facets of working with defined groups of individuals. The scientist might also have worked with animal models and studies of various kinds, or human experimental cellular models. All these approaches have in common a prospective aspect, where you set out with perhaps a team, to uncover every aspect of the problem as far as possible through planning and design, whilst using relatively predictable experimental platforms to understand and interpret the mechanisms of action or toxicity of a particular agent. These mechanisms can thus be tracked from the cellular level, right through to tissues, organs and finally to the whole organism, be it human or animal. Whilst rats, mice and cellular systems are of course more controllable than patients or volunteers, generally, the operators of these models have a relatively stable platform to work with which has been evolved or designed so that others in their field can compare and interpret the results and apply them to their own situation if needs be.

The world of occupational toxicity at first appears to be fairly straightforward; there is a toxic agent or agents, and there are individuals reporting certain specific effects. However, there, the similarities with a scientist or clinical practitioner's known world can end. There is no immediately apparent 'control' that the professional can exert over the process of toxicity which has already happened and must be teased out, from a morass of conflicting information from the employer, the claimant, the claimant's nearest and dearest, as well as the claimant's work colleagues. The would-be report writer has to try to draw out a consistent picture of what happened, in terms of timelines of exposure, degree of exposure, routes of exposure, elements of provided protection, elements of the worker's knowledge of the risks, the degree they should have been informed of those risks and, ultimately, who is likely to be telling the unvarnished truth.

Incidentally, if you were perhaps to become interested in carrying out occupational toxicity clinical work, report writing experience might give you a perspective as to why several apparently obvious conditions related to occupation are not always accepted as attributable to occupation by the medical profession, government organisations or, indeed, other scientists. This is probably because most occupational toxicity investigations are retrospective, rather than prospective, so there is rarely an opportunity to plan an investigation with adequate controls and sufficient resources to determine all the factors involved. Even a retrospective study will be fraught with problems, ranging from finding appropriate controls, to sorting out all the confounding variables, such as what agents were involved, degree of exposure, establishing which workplace activities are related to exposure and myriad other factors. There is also the issue as to who would pay for such work; certainly, the companies involved are unlikely to fund it, and governments or regulatory agencies cannot be expected to foot the bill either. On a darker and somewhat conspiratorial note, it has been suggested that perhaps it is in nobody's interests except the victims of occupational health damage that such definitive studies go ahead, as they might trigger large numbers of compensation claims which, given the slippery record of some industries such as that of asbestos, will be laid eventually at the door of the taxpayer. Ironically, the truth is often more prosaic; in the late 1990s, many claims were submitted for some organophosphate-related injuries, and the courts felt that the quality of the causation evidence was so poor that pilot studies were commissioned and funded to cast light on the issue. Indeed, it was agreed that the cases should be put on hold until the outcome of the studies became known. Perhaps predictably, the findings of the study were inconclusive, and this area is still under intensive study which is outlined in more detail in Chapter 5.

Back to the causality report: this conforms closely with the standard required for a manuscript to be submitted to a good-quality journal, in terms of precision and clarity of language, organisation and referencing. However, it is by no means the 'final word' on the case, in the way a peer-reviewed and published paper might be on a clinical trial or a series of experiments. The causality report is essentially a 'best view': an opinion based on detailed knowledge of mechanisms, examination of the presented evidence, scientific and otherwise, as well as the 'balance of probabilities' that the claimant is telling the truth. So it could be said that the causality report is part of the whole process of a claimant seeking redress, which is summarised in Figure 2.1, but not necessarily the definitive part; the decisions are ultimately made by the legal teams on the behest of the employer as well as the claimant and, in the last resort, the court.

The next chapters provide some case histories which demonstrate the diversity and complexity of some claimant's experiences of occupational health issues as well as my own attempts at exploring them in my reports. It has to be emphasised that causality report writing is an evolving and very subjective process, and you effectively learn as you progress through different cases. Fictional forensic entertainment usually features the manifestation of an appropriate 'smoking gun' around 45 min into an hour-long show to provide enough time for a suitably blazing and percussive dénouement. Unfortunately, this does not happen often in reality, and if there had been an obvious clear path to the truth in a case, it would probably have been settled long before the stage of consulting prospective report writers.

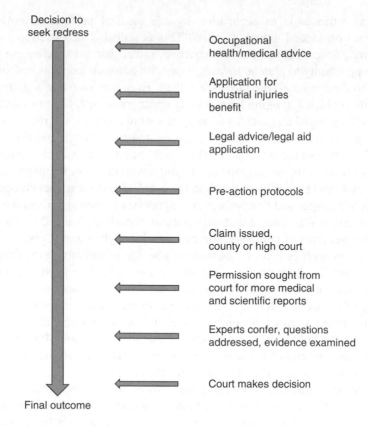

Figure 2.1 Summarised pathway from the claimant's initial position, towards seeking some form of recognition of injury, as well as financial redress, beginning with an application for day-to-day support from the Department of Work and Pensions Industrial Injuries Benefit Scheme. Irrespective of the benefit decision, the claimant might then pursue their case through the legal system.

References

1. Greater Manchester Hazards Centre, Windrush Millennium Centre, 70 Alexandra Road Manchester M16 7WD, 0161 636 7557, mail@gmhazards.org.uk; www.gmhazards.org.uk (accessed on 11 November 2013).
2. Sheffield Occupational Health Advisory Service (SOHAS), 4th Floor Furnival House, 48 Furnival Gate, Sheffield S1 4QP, 0114 275 5760, sohas@sohas.co.uk; www.sohas.co.uk (accessed on 11 November 2013).
3. London Hazards Centre, Hampstead Town Hall Centre, 213 Haverstock Hill, London NW3 4QP, 020 7794 5999, mail@lhc.org.uk; www.lhc.org.uk (accessed on 11 November 2013)
4. West Midlands Hazards Trust, 138 Digbeth, Birmingham, B5 6DR, 0121 678 8853, www.asbestossupportwm.org; www.hazardscampaign.org.uk/direct/dirp12629.htm (accessed on 11 November 2013).

5. Industrial Injuries Disablement Benefit. www.gov.uk/industrial-injuries-disablement-benefit/eligibility, Appendix 1: List of diseases covered by Industrial Injuries Disablement Benefit: www.dwp.gov.uk/publications/specialist-guides/technical-guidance/db1-a-guide-to-industrial-injuries/appendix/appendix-1/ (accessed on 11 November 2013).

6. Ministry of Justice Civil Procedure Rules 2013. www.justice.gov.uk/courts/procedure-rules/civil/forms (accessed on 11 November 2013).

7. Legal Aid Agency. http://www.justice.gov.uk/about/laa; www.gov.uk/legal-aid/eligibility; www.justice.gov.uk/legal-aid/assess-your-clients-eligibility (accessed on 11 November 2013).

8. Ministry of Justice: Civil Procedure Rules, Pre-Action Protocol for Disease and Illness Claims. http://www.justice.gov.uk/courts/procedure-rules/civil/protocol/prot_dis (accessed on 11 November 2013).

9. Ministry of Justice: Queen's Bench Guide. www.justice.gov.uk/downloads/courts/queens-bench/queen-bench-guide.pdf (accessed 14 May 2013.

10. ATSDR (Agency for toxic substances and disease registry), 1,1,1-trichloroethane. http://www.atsdr.cdc.gov/tfacts70.pdf (accessed on 11 November 2013).

11. COUNCIL DIRECTIVE 1999/13/EC of 11 March 1999 on the limitation of emissions of volatile organic compounds due to the use of organic solvents in certain activities and installations. http://eur-lex.europa.eu/LexUriServ/LexUriServ.do?uri=OJ:L:1999:085:0001:0001:EN:PDF (accessed on 11 November 2013).

12. Doll R, Hill, AB. The mortality of doctors in relation to their smoking habits: a preliminary report. BMJ 228, 1451–1455, 1954.

3
Acute toxicity: Case histories of solvent exposure

3.1 Introduction

Assessing the effect of toxins on the human body in a 'real world' context can be problematic. Often, the action of a toxin is conveniently termed either 'acute' or 'chronic'. Whilst medically, acute effects are usually taken to be an impact on the body over minutes to hours, for the purposes of occupational toxicity, I have been very broad in my use of the term, to distinguish short-term chemical effects, such as solvent intoxication, from chronic impacts which lead to permanent and life-threatening conditions such as cancer or other forms of debilitation, which will be discussed in the next chapter. This is not to say that acute toxicity cannot cause permanent and life-threatening injury; rather, it is a convenient separation of the two types of cases I will describe. In an occupational context, it is possible to suffer acute toxicity, for minutes or hours per day, over many months or even years. You could perhaps say that the person is essentially enduring 'chronic acute' toxicity. Their exposure might not be every day, but often enough for the toxic agent to either accumulate in terms of its residence in the body, or its toxic effects may make a serious impact on the worker's physical or mental health, or both in some cases. The individual may be able to withstand the toxicity for some time, but eventually, their resilience is overcome, and they start to suffer health consequences. You might think that if you were in this situation, you would refuse to carry on working in a toxic environment, hurling down your tools and confronting management with the reality of such unreasonable conditions. This does happen, but often workers seem to endure work environments which are hostile to their health for long periods until they are made so ill that they actually cannot physically continue to do the job.

There are many factors that conspire to prevent workers objecting or speaking out against their work conditions. Most of us are familiar with the idea that we should 'tough it out', perhaps with regard to a cold virus or 'flu', or a minor injury. Whilst this attitude makes an employee appear industrious and dependable, in some cases, coupled with ignorance or lack of realisation of the progressively serious impact a

Expert Report Writing in Toxicology: Forensic, Scientific and Legal Aspects,
First Edition. Michael D. Coleman.
© 2014 John Wiley & Sons, Ltd. Published 2014 by John Wiley & Sons, Ltd.

toxin is having, it can lead to a health catastrophe. Exposure to many chemicals such as solvents, as well as toxic fumes related to welding, for example, can sometimes have effects which are similar to the onset of a minor respiratory illness, such as in the case of the well-documented condition of weld fume fever. Few of us possess highly specialised knowledge outside of our interests or occupations, so it is unreasonable to expect an employee to be familiar with the detailed effects of the agents they are working with, particularly for the first time of exposure, unless the employer supplies appropriate information through their 'duty of care' obligations. You might also expect that the average employee trusts their employer not to expose them to something injurious, so even in the face of progressive evidence of toxicity and debilitation, he or she might 'soldier on'.

Another issue, perhaps more applicable to males, is the somewhat 'macho' aspect to physical work in that it really should be hard, dirty and tough and even contain an element of danger. Whilst anyone who has been down a mine is impressed by the physicality of the work and the unpleasantness of the environment, miners were often proud of how they endured their working lifetime, and consequently they saw themselves as an elite amongst working men. Hence, when the pits closed in the United Kingdom, from the 1970s onwards, incalculably more was lost, other than just paid employment.

Another factor can be the degree of usage of available protective measures; even the casual observer today might sometimes see men in various working environments, as they disdain protective equipment. Grinding, welding, cutting, sawing and hammering may occur through showers of sparks and shards of flying metal without a sign of any mask, visor or even gloves. It is still possible to watch men on building sites or in road works cutting or drilling without apparent ear protection, and the noise is shattering 30 yards away. These attitudes, coupled with a conspicuous failure on the part of some employers to take seriously their duty of care, can lead the creation of working environments which even today are extremely difficult to endure for more than a short period, without some impact on health.

This chapter will describe case histories where toxins have caused acute, as well as 'chronic acute' effects on worker's health. Solvents are a convenient example of agents, which can, in effect, repeatedly poison an individual over hours, days and even months of exposure. Some element of recovery occurs during the intervening periods of non-exposure, but gradually and sometimes almost imperceptibly, serious physical and mental health consequences may arise. The following sections outline the scale and variety of solvent usage, followed by their particular properties which promote their toxic effects, as well as the difficulties encountered in discerning the long-term impact of these chemicals on an exposed individual.

3.2 Solvents in adhesives

Modern manufacturing techniques have automated many processes, such as car and electrical goods manufacture. Obviously, such technology has made a vast difference to the health of workforces around the world, as exposure to toxic vapours of various kinds is progressively minimised and machines can function efficiently in the most hostile of environments. The disadvantage for societies requiring high numbers of unskilled jobs is that far fewer people are employed in automated premises and those that are, are most likely to be high-skill individuals needed to maintain software systems and machines. Despite these advances, many of our most basic possessions, such as furniture, shoes and leather goods, are still to some extent assembled largely by hand, using manufactured components. Like all industries, operations proceed on the basis of minimising labour costs, which are by far the greatest component of their turnover, hence, these industries can be concentrated where labour is cheap and workers' rights are few. Interestingly, such hand-build processes can also operate in small, speciality industries in developed countries, such as bespoke leather products related to horse riding, speciality shoes or custom furniture manufacture.

All these assembly processes have relied on adhesives of various types for centuries. Thousands of years before the birth of Christ, ancient cultures were repairing pots and other domestic wares with adhesives based on waste animal, fish or vegetable material, which were quite useful, but very time-consuming to produce, involving considerable boiling and processing. They also had their limitations in their applicability and effectiveness. By the early part of the twentieth century, various synthetic adhesives and sealers appeared, such as phenol and urea formaldehydes, which were followed by acrylic epoxy resins in the 1930s and the ubiquitous cyanoacrylates in the 1950s. Since then, adhesive and sealing technology has burgeoned to provide products which can suit any manufacturing process, providing practically instant bonding with maximum strength to facilitate rapid volume manufacture. To achieve this, the adhesives depend on a battery of different organic solvents, which are required to evaporate rapidly to assist with adhesive curing and bonding. Inevitably, to cut costs, adhesives used were based on readily available organic solvents such as the alkanes, like hexane, and aromatic solvents, such as toluene and xylene. There are dozens of other solvents in use in industry, ranging from the various methyl ketones to haloalkanes and many different ether derivatives. However, with one or two exceptions, the very properties which make solvents highly desirable in manufacturing are the reason they are toxic to those that work with them.

3.3   Solvent toxicity

The toxicity of solvents depends on three factors: firstly, their volatility, secondly, their lipophilicity and finally, their individual routes of metabolism that are intended to clear them from the body. Solvent volatility is demonstrated to all of us at some point in our daily lives, when we might become aware of the strong smell of petrol when filling up the car, or when in a confined space, a nail polish remover is used or an adhesive is applied. If you have worked with different solvents, you can recognise their odours. Perhaps I should not admit to a favourite organic solvent, but a

colleague used methyl tertiary butyl ether for many months in an adjacent laboratory to mine, and I used to recognise it in petrol in the United States through its
rather pleasant but strong menthol-like odour. It was introduced to promote better
combustion of fuels to improve emissions, but it is less popular now that it has been
shown to accumulate in groundwater. Solvent volatility means that in a confined
space, quite high concentrations of the solvent will enter the atmosphere within a
few seconds of release from a vessel.

The second property the solvents possess is their lipophilicity, which means that
they can both dissolve oils and dissolve in oils. This is useful when they act as
degreasers in many industries, as well as when they act as a vehicle for hydrophobic
adhesive mixes. Since our lungs have a very high surface area and the alveoli have
lipids in their membranes, this means we absorb volatile solvents very quickly
indeed and they proceed through our blood to the brain in just a few seconds. The
brain is highly lipophilic, and the blood brain barrier, a special property of the blood
vessels that supply the brain which protects it from various water-soluble toxins,
is no barrier to solvents. This means that these chemicals enter and affect the brain
in a similar manner to that of surgical anaesthetics. So most solvents in sufficient
concentrations can cause drowsiness, followed by mental befuddlement and impairment of reflexes leading to progressive incapacitation of mental performance and
awareness, until eventually unconsciousness and death occurs in very high concentrations of the agent. Occasionally, tragedies still happen when workers are overcome by fumes in solvent tanks during repair processes, and their colleagues can
meet the same fate if they try to rescue them without breathing equipment. A friend
of mine once laid a tile floor in his house on a warm day using a powerful adhesive.
He began to notice that the tiles were bending and curling, and he tried very hard
to flatten them out. He was later found unconscious by his wife and when he
had recovered as he inspected the half-inch-thick rigid tiles, he realised that the
'tile curling' was actually an extraordinarily vivid hallucination. By the 1980s and
1990s, it was realised that adequate extraction systems were necessary to prevent
solvents intoxicating workers and even gradually incapacitating them after several
hours' exposure to a particular agent. More recently, even volatile solvents in
domestic paints are being removed in favour of water or heavier alcohols, partly in
response to the toxicity of solvents and their environmental impact, but also due to
their widespread abuse.

There is a third issue with solvents, which is specific to individual agents, where
a solvent exerts a perhaps unique toxic effect, which can be related to how the liver
eliminates it from the body, and this can make it more dangerous than other agents.
The alkane n-hexane is one good example of this. In the shoe industry in the 1960s
and 1970s in several countries, many workers were found to be suffering from a
particular type of neuronal damage, known as peripheral neuropathy. This condition
begins with numbness and progresses gradually to paralysis of the arms, hands and
feet. It was eventually associated with exposure to high concentrations (500–2000 ppm)
of the n-hexane in poorly ventilated premises for at least 6 months, but more often
several years. Interestingly, the workers did usually recover, but this process was

very gradual and often not complete within 2 years of diagnosis [1, 2]. Some residual debilitation resulted, and in some cases, the optic nerve was also affected. The mechanism of action was not hexane itself, but rather a metabolite formed by the liver in its efforts to remove this solvent from the body, known as 2,5-hexanedione. This is a neurotoxin which acts on peripheral, rather than central nervous system (CNS) neurones, by cross-linking structural proteins within neurones, which supply the muscles of the arms, legs and hands. This effect is highly specific to the 2,5 derivative and does not happen with other closely related hexanediones, such as the 2,3 and 3,4 derivatives, which are actually food flavourings, although they do display some toxicity which is unrelated to that of the 2,5 derivative [3]. Hence, hexane has a deserved reputation for causing neurological toxicity and its usage is generally discouraged in adhesives. Incredibly, as late as 2008, workers assembling touchscreens for Apple computers in China were told to use hexane as it evaporated more rapidly than alcohols, so the production process could be accelerated [4]. Sadly, the workers soon reported the classic symptoms as described above. Hence, manufacturers have striven to either reduce hexane usage or replace it with related isomers or other alkanes which are not associated with peripheral toxicity.

3.4   The real-world confusion of symptoms

When an individual develops a symptom or a series of symptoms which affect their lives to the point that they seek medical attention, the doctor will listen to the account of the symptoms, perhaps examine the patient and then consider a range of possible diagnoses and subsequent treatments. If a patient reports a series of respiratory-based symptoms, these might be connected with asthma or other long-standing conditions. Patients also bring their own habits to the situation, such as smoking, drinking and illicit drug intake, which they may or may not be entirely honest about. There are many causes of exacerbation of respiratory tract problems, and regarding the CNS, several conditions can lead to nausea and dizziness, headaches and general feelings of tiredness, as well as changes in mood and attitude. Solvents are capable of causing all these effects, although many other explanations can also apply, ranging from migraines, various infections, as well as complex alcohol and prescription/illicit drug combination actions. Hence, the situation is far from clear; if the doctor does not ask what the patient does for a living, then he is likely to try to find an explanation for the symptoms in terms of well-known diseases and conditions, and/or some of the patient's activities of which he is actually aware. If he or she does ask about the patient's occupation, then there is a possibility that the diagnosis could be skewed towards a list of known effects of a particular process or agent, perhaps discounting other causes. Alternatively, as mentioned elsewhere, the patient may have already found a list of problems associated with a particular agent or process, and they, or their spouse, may have 'decided' that the occupation is to blame, and they will pursue this idea to its bitter end. In many cases, not knowing or meeting the individual before his symptoms of, say excessive aggression or anger, means that it is virtually impossible to prove that the person is acting out of character, except for the testimony of friends and colleagues, who may have their own reasons for supporting the individual's claim that they were seriously and permanently impaired by their occupation.

Hence, in many cases, a series of arguments can be forwarded over the causality of a particular set of symptoms based on the description provided by the claimant or a medical report, yet there is still considerable doubt as to whether the occupational circumstances are really to blame for the situation. In the case histories in this chapter, it is apparent that the degree of certainty that can be ascribed to a particular explanation appears to unfortunately lie in the severity of the symptoms and experience of the claimant, and even then, other explanations can be provided. Other situations, where the impact on the claimant's life is not quite so intense, are even more difficult to accurately ascribe causation.

3.5   Case histories: General format

The following case histories illustrate the impact of solvent exposure on several individuals. As outlined in Chapter 2, when a report is submitted, a list of cited references would be included at the end of the document. In this book, all references quoted in the case reports and in the text are listed at the end of each chapter for convenience. In addition, again as mentioned in Chapter 2, all reports are required to contain a brief resume of the expert's qualifications and suitability for the task, as well as the declaration from the Queen's Bench Guide over the duty of the expert to assist the court. Those sections are included in Section 3.6 for demonstration purposes, but are omitted from all subsequent cases in this book, for reasons of brevity.

3.6   Case history 1: Mr A and volatile petroleum mixture exposure

Mr A was a 42-year-old skilled worker in the field of leather product manufacture, making items such as saddles and bridles, having served an apprenticeship in this area. He joined a new company and worked in a small room without extraction facilities using various adhesives, where the only window was barred and inaccessible. No personal protective equipment was issued to him. After only 6 weeks in this particular job, he suffered an acute psychological crisis on the way home one day, when he actually abandoned his motorcycle 'due to feelings of invincibility' and euphoria and curiously was even anxious to destroy his helmet so he could not use his motorcycle. Although he found his way home, the scale of his irrationality led his wife to take him to hospital, and his psychological state was so profoundly disordered that the psychiatric crisis team considered sectioning him. After a week or so in hospital, his recovery was protracted, due to several psychological problems, including panic attacks, coupled with a lack of sleep, paranoia and general anxiety. He was unable to work for several months, and on the basis of medical advice from those who had treated him that his condition was almost certainly linked with his work, he sought legal advice on gaining some form of redress for his ordeal. Medical reports were commissioned on the state of his health when he started proceedings, and a causation report was sought from myself over the possible link with the solvent bases of the adhesives and his acute psychological and physical crises. I was furnished with all his medical records, as well as the medical reports submitted as part of the case.

*RE: An Expert Report prepared for Birmingham Crown Court by Dr M.D. Coleman on the instructions of **** Litigation concerning the case of Mr A (Claimant) against **** Saddlemakers (defendants).*

Expert qualifications

I am Dr Michael Damian Coleman, and I am the holder of a Doctorate in Biochemical Pharmacology from the University of Liverpool. I received my first degree in Pharmacology (Class I) from the same University. I received my Ph.D. in 1985 and won a Scholarship against international competition to study in the Division of Experimental Therapeutics of the Walter Reed Army Institute of Research at Washington D.C. from 1986 to 1988. This Institute is one of the premier research organisations in the United States. On my return to the United Kingdom, I was awarded a Wellcome Fellowship in Toxicology, again in competition with other scientists. I have published over 84 full scientific papers, review articles and scientific meeting abstracts on various aspects of Pharmacology and Toxicology. I have studied the behaviour of aromatic compounds in human systems for many years. This necessitates a thorough understanding of the chemistry and biology of these agents and how they damage the human body. In addition, I have developed strategies whereby these toxicities can be reduced or avoided completely. Currently, I lecture on the subjects of Toxicology and Pharmacology at Aston University to Pharmacy and Human Biology Students. I am consulted locally, nationally and internationally on Biochemical Toxicology, and I am a member of the British Toxicology Society.

Material instructions

Mr A contends that his exposure to a variety of different petro-chemical products encountered as part of his job at **** Saddlemakers caused him to develop severe psychological disturbances, which subsequently necessitated hospitalisation. I have been requested to provide an expert report on whether Mr A's condition can be causatively linked with his occupation and the implications for his future employment and quality of life.

Nature and consequences of solvent exposure

Introduction

Different solvents are known to exhibit specific central (CNS: brain and spinal cord) and peripheral (nerves in the rest of the body) neurological effects. To link the neurological symptoms Mr A suffered with the solvents involved, it is necessary to establish the nature of the solvent exposure, which may be sub-divided as the type of solvent(s) involved and the extent of exposure.

Type of solvents

1. There is a minor terminological confusion over the exact solvent contents of the adhesives employed by Mr A. The Excel safety data sheet lists the main solvent mix as 'hexane mixture of isomers, 60–100%'. Later on, **** Saddlemakers list C30 as supplied by Crispin, as Howstik 129, which was 5% *n*-hexane and 30–60% naphtha. Effectively, they may be the same thing, as the adhesive solvent content appears very similar as obtained from two suppliers. Either way, the description is still imprecise as the exact solvent combination is not clear. In my experience, other manufacturers do list the precise solvent contents of their lacquers/adhesives and include the percentage proportions.

2. Reading from the Crispin data sheet, Howstik 129 (C30) is based on a maximum of 5% *n*-hexane and 30–60% naphtha, which I take to be a mixture of light branched and straight chain aliphatic hydrocarbons, similar to hexane, which are stated to have been desulphurised, and all the aromatic agents removed, probably by solvent extraction or hydrogenation. It is assumed that the remainder of the C30 mixture contains the resin components which provide the bonding properties of the adhesive. The other adhesive system is Solibond PAJ, which lists a solvent mixture of hexane isomers, again including not more than 5% *n*-hexane itself. Again, it is not clear exactly what this mixture is. Its density is given as 0.72–0.75, and the flashpoint is listed as −26°C. *n*-Hexane itself has a lower density, but a similar flashpoint.

3. A close commercially available relative of the solvent mixture used in C30 is broadly similar to a Shell product, such as SBP 60/95 LNH (www.shell.com; density 0.7, flashpoint −25°C). This special boiling point solvent mixture is a C6–C7 hydrocarbon mix, with less than 3% *n*-hexane, and is made from hydrogenated feedstock and is thus very low (<0.01%) in aromatic hydrocarbons. These types of solvents are used in many industries as bases for many different adhesives. In general, aromatic hydrocarbons are associated with CNS effects, while *n*-hexane is a very well-documented peripheral nervous system toxin. The minimisation of these substances in solvent mixtures is already known to be important by manufacturers and end-users, and this is reflected in the low contents of these two toxins in C30 and solibond PAJ and the Shell product.

4. The Road Transport Information in the safety data sheet for the C30 solvent mix is identical to that of the Shell product. In summary, it is likely that the solvents that Mr A breathed on a daily basis would have been *n*-hexane, C6–C7 aliphatic light paraffins, some branched and some straight chain, as well as some heavier paraffins. The lighter fractions, C6–C8 would exert a vapour pressure similar to components of unleaded petrol, although unlike petrol, the aromatic contents of the solvent mixtures are likely to be so small as to be negligible toxicologically.

5. Mr A mentioned that he was also exposed to a 'stronger' glue, called C25, which dried much more quickly than C30, approximately 14 days before his psychotic episode. To date, no information has been obtained on the nature of the solvent mix for this product. Indeed, **** Saddlemakers deny in their letter dated September 11 any knowledge of this adhesive's existence or its use on their premises. Therefore, I feel it would be unwise to speculate on the content of 'C25' or its possible effects.

Extent of exposure

1. The data sheet for C30 warns that it should only be used in areas which are well ventilated, and local exhaust ventilation should be present. Goggles, respirator and protective gloves should be used. Respiratory protection should be used if level in the air exceeds the occupational exposure standards, which are listed as long-term exposure, 8 h at 500 ppm, and short-term exposure, 15 min at 1000 ppm. The saturated vapour concentration of the Shell solvent was listed as equivalent to 718 ppm. As the Shell product is similar in its properties to the solvent base of C30, it could be assumed that in a room without any ventilation at approximately normal room temperature (25 °C), the solvent base of C30 would reach saturation in the atmosphere at a value similar to that of the Shell solvent.

2. Mr A was apparently using 5 L of the adhesive every week in a poorly ventilated small room, so it is not surprising that the stated 500 ppm value for chronic exposure to C30 would have been comfortably exceeded during the average working day. In warm weather, when the air temperature would exceed 25°C, exposure would probably increase, even allowing for the effects of a rise in humidity.

Consequences of exposure

1. Volatile solvents are designed to carry an adhesive or paint and, due to their high vapour pressure, evaporate rapidly and leave minimal residue. Most people are familiar with the range of evaporation necessary in solvents, from aromatics in gloss paints, which may take days to dry, to glues and adhesives, such as epoxy resins, which are solid within minutes. Adhesives must cure very quickly; hence, these agents contain the most volatile solvents which evaporate most readily. Therefore, the most desirable property of volatile solvents makes them extremely hazardous in the workplace. Often, a long period of exposure to a solvent can effectively inhibit the ability of the individual to smell it. This further erodes the worker's perception of his exposure, notwithstanding the toxicity they are causing in the process.

2. Organic solvents cause two main types of toxicity: to the skin and to the CNS. They are very effective as de-fatting agents, and this usually leads to dermatitis in most individuals if exposure is high enough. The volatility of the solvents enables them to enter the lungs and become absorbed into the bloodstream within minutes. Solvents can then reach the brain within 3–5 min, and they enter the fatty areas of the membranes of the brain cells. Although it is not fully understood how they actually disrupt neural tissue, they cause a well-defined series of symptoms, which include disorientation, euphoria, giddiness and confusion [5]. It is well established that n-hexane will cause damage to the peripheral nervous system, which can be manifested as problems of movement of the hands and feet, as well as tingling sensations and loss of feeling.

3. This is because the body chemically converts the solvent to a specifically neuro-toxic metabolite, 2,5-hexanedione. This process has been known since the early 1960s in the shoemaking and laminating industries, so consequently, levels of n-hexane have been maintained at a low level in solvent combinations since then [6]. Reading Mr A's case history, I have not seen any mention of peripheral neu-ropathy, so despite the presence of n-hexane and his undoubted exposure to this neurotoxin, it was fortunately not of sufficient concentration to cause any apparent damage to the nerves of his extremities.

4. In general, aliphatic solvents such as the agents which make up the solvent that Mr A used in his work are known to be responsible for a number of conditions when exposure is chronic. These include weight loss, anaemia, proteinuria, haematuria and bone marrow hypoplasia [5]. Other symptoms include euphoria, fatigue, anxiety, irritability, headaches, depression, behavioural changes and cognitive disorders [7].

5. Mr A exhibited most of these symptoms, such as proteinuria (a well-established marker of renal damage) and the loss of two stone in weight in the 3 months prior to his admission to hospital. His behavioural and mood changes also appeared to be consistent with chronic aliphatic solvent exposure. The yellowing of the skin may have been jaundice, while the skin 'elasticity' is associated with severe dehydration. These features are those of individuals who habitually abuse organic solvents.

6. If the yellowing was jaundice, this would be connected with the general disruption to liver function which can be caused when it metabolises some chemicals to toxic metabolites, which can damage the liver. Mrs A reported that a sample of his semen was orange/yellow coloured. This might be linked with the jaundice. Although there are no supplied details, Mr A was apparently suffering from overproduction of 'acid', which was attributed to his liver. In the absence of more information, this could be assumed to be metabolic acidosis, which can arise from a variety of toxic conditions or excess formation of uric acid, which is normally associated with gout. It is perplexing that amongst the biochemical tests carried out on Mr A, only creatinine clearance was higher than normal limits.

7. High creatinine clearance is another parameter associated with kidney damage, and it is likely that when Mr A was admitted to hospital, his creatinine values may have been much higher and his kidney function may have been impaired. The tests

supplied in the medical notes appear to have been conducted at or around September 1, more than 2 weeks after Mr A's crisis became manifest. It is certain that in that period of time, the solvents and their metabolites would have been cleared fully from his system (aided by his high fluid intake during his hospitalisation), and it would be likely that his liver function would have recovered.

8. Bone marrow hypoplasia usually means that the marrow shrinks and is less able to make immune cells which can thus predispose the victim to infection. In general, aromatic solvents are more CNS toxic than aliphatic solvents [7], although in the case of Mr A, his level of chronic exposure has been so high that the normally less toxic aliphatic compounds have exerted a potent effect on his brain function.

A possible link between symptoms and solvent exposure

The range of Mr A's neurobehavioral symptoms is certainly wide and might be interpreted to be indicative of a form of latent paranoid psychosis. Dr X, an internationally known clinical expert, of the Poisons Unit at City Hospital described them as 'florid'. Some of the symptoms appear consistent with schizophrenic symptoms, and it could be argued that he may have developed this crisis at any time, and the solvent exposure may not be related to his condition. However, I believe that on balance, this is not the case for the following reasons:

1. In general, schizophrenic symptoms appear early in young adult life, usually from the age 16+. It is unusual for these symptoms to appear for the first time in an individual at the age of around 40.

2. Mr A has experienced panic attacks previously, although this was in response to an acute emotional crisis, that is, his wife threatening to leave him in 1997. At the time of his psychotic episode in August 2000, he was apparently not under any specific strain, emotional or financial.

3. When solvent abusers are hospitalised to 'dry out', the symptoms they present are similar to those of Mr A, a mixture of physical problems due to the toxicity of the solvents to the liver, and psychiatric issues caused by chronic solvent damage caused in the brain, which can take months to resolve, if it does at all.

4. The course of Mr A's recovery from his episode is not compatible with an acute exposure to aliphatic solvents, which is usually confusion and narcosis, which would wear off in hours as the solvents were exhaled and metabolised. If his exposure had been purely acute, he would have been more likely to recover as a person might from a hangover.

5. Although many of Mr A's symptoms appeared consistent with schizophrenia, he demonstrated a consistent degree of insight and awareness of his condition, which is usually conspicuously lacking in persons suffering from a true schizophrenic episode.

6. No medication has been necessary in Mr A's case, and he has not displayed similar symptoms almost 2 years after his first episode. If his condition was a latent

psychosis unrelated to solvents, it would be more likely that he would have suffered at least one other episode since.

7. Many documented clinical experiences with chronic solvent abusers are rather similar to Mr A's exposure to high solvent concentrations during his work routine. Psychosis due to chronic solvent abuse is associated with general symptoms such as hallucination, delusions and thought disturbances [8]. Other symptoms have been described, such as incoherence, delusions of persecution and control, although in one study, individuals suffering many of these symptoms maintained good emotional contact with each other; those authors maintained that the symptoms of solvent psychosis differ from schizophrenia [9]. The general pattern of Mr A's experience, I believe, bears many similarities with the effects of chronic exposure to volatile solvents encountered during the course of his work, rather than a latent psychosis.

Long-term consequences for Mr A

1. Exposure to solvents on a long-term basis can result in a neurotoxic syndrome known as chronic toxic encephalopathy (CTE). Symptoms can range from impairment of short-term memory and learning skills, to increased irritability, tiredness, sleeping problems and changes in personality [10, 11]. Follow-up studies have shown that once removed from the solvent-laden environment, persistent deficits can be observed in persons who were severely affected initially [7]. In Dr L's letter to Dr S, of January 19, more than 5 months after the psychotic episode, he did state that Mrs A 'still expressed some concerns regarding his mental health'. In Mrs A's statement, made in December of this year, she writes that 'my husband appears to be better now'. She did not state that he was recovered or fully recovered. Her wording implies that she still at that point harboured anxieties over Mr A's health.

2. His medical notes indicate that in terms of general physical and mental well-being, it has been concluded that he is fully recovered from his condition. If this is the case, then he is relatively fortunate to escape without a permanent neurological deficit, although I feel that the extent of any lasting neurobiological damage that the solvents may have inflicted on Mr A should be determined by professional evaluation of his short-term memory capacity and memory span, as well as his learning and cognitive abilities.

Mr A's future capacity for work

1. It is not clear at this stage whether solvent exposure has caused permanent neurological deficits in Mr A resulting in changes to his personality, as well as his ability to learn and retain new tasks and procedures. It is apparent that his physical health is recovered. The type of neurological problems that can occur after medium/long-term solvent exposure would adversely affect his ability to retain a job which was commensurate with his pre-exposure capabilities. It is clear that Mr A's earning potential has been eroded since his crisis, and this situation continues. His living standards and those of his family have been reduced through no fault of their own.

Overall, it is apparent that Mr A's career prospects, the quality of his personal and family life, as well as their material and emotional expectations have all been damaged as a consequence of his occupation.

Summary

In my opinion, the balance of probabilities is that Mr A's exposure to a mixture of aliphatic hydrocarbon solvents was substantially greater than recommended limits for a considerable period of time. This chronic exposure to neurotoxic agents caused gradual changes in his behaviour and general health until a severe crisis point was reached in August 2000. It is still not certain whether the solvent exposure has permanently affected Mr A's mental health.

Declaration

I understand that my duty is to help the court on matters within my expertise, namely Biochemical Toxicology. This duty to the court overrides any obligations to the person from whom instructions or payment have been received. In writing this report, I have complied with this duty, and I believe the facts I have stated herein are true and the opinions I have expressed are correct.

M.D. Coleman, Ph.D.

3.6.1 Case comment

Mr A eventually recovered more than 6 months after his hospitalisation, and although he had worked in the leather finishing trade for many years, the only job he was able to accept was as a mail sorter. This meant that his income dropped considerably, and he was unable to use his skills in a job that he did not enjoy. The Health and Safety Executive inspected the Saddlemakers' premises and served an improvement notice on them regarding ventilation and personal protection issues, and they did leave those premises soon after. Mr A was given an undisclosed financial settlement, although it appeared at the time unlikely that even a generous settlement could compensate for his loss of his livelihood.

The report discussed the suggestion that Mr A's symptoms could have been accounted for by some form of either schizophrenic or even bipolar depression 'manic phase' of behaviour, as many of the facets of his emotional state and mood are described by sufferers of these conditions. However, as mentioned in the report, these mental illnesses surface usually on the threshold of adult life, and it is exceedingly rare for them to appear during what is effectively early middle age, without any previous warning signs. In addition, such conditions once manifest reappear regularly, and this did not occur with Mr A. There were no other alcohol or drugs-of-abuse 'skeletons' in Mr A's closet, so to speak, which might have precipitated a severe psychosis. In addition, conditions such as schizophrenia and bipolar disorder do not generally have the many physical organ-related problems that Mr A reported, and the combination of his symptoms, circumstances and the lack of repetition of the effects since suggests that the cause was indeed long-term intoxication with aliphatic solvent vapours.

In retrospect, it might seem surprising that Mr A could have withstood such a high concentration of these vapours for so long without question or at least some attempt to improve his working environment. However, solvents have complex mood-enhancing effects on the brain, and the evidence suggests that he was in effect 'blissfully' unaware of his degree of chronic intoxication. It is sobering that an individual's occupation could effectively make him parallel the experience of a solvent abuser, without any practical insight into the source of his mood enhancement, or any awareness of the risks of the major psychological trauma that he was to endure.

3.7   Case history 2: Mr B and dichloromethane exposure

The toxicity of hexane and its intense flammability have led to the use of many other solvents in the adhesive industry, although the substitute solvents are hardly an improvement. As mentioned in Chapter 2, chlorinated solvents are used in large quantities in industrial processes, and one of their advantages is their lack of flammability compared with other hydrocarbon solvents, although the sweet-smelling carbon tetrachloride I used in school chemistry practicals is a known hepatotoxin and is not used in adhesives. Dichloromethane (DCM), however, is a component of several adhesives, and it has a strong minty vapour. It is also very dense, and bottles of the stuff are noticeably heavier compared with those of other solvents. Whilst it is not really flammable *per se*, it can demonstrate a crackling/sparking effect in a flame, and it is capable of causing explosions in high oxygen levels. The following case recalls Mr B, who worked for a Company that made furniture. His daily duties involved working in a booth using several adhesives to assemble kitchen units, and in contrast to the previous case, he did not suffer from a life-changing incapacitating experience; rather, he endured a series of more subtle and chronic psychological effects.

The turning point was probably when Mr B discovered a data sheet on the main adhesive he was using, and it listed a series of possible toxic effects related to DCM, which he felt were alarmingly similar to his own experience. He refused to continue using this adhesive, and his medical problems did appear to ease, although his symptoms of depression did not immediately disappear. He quit his job soon afterwards, and the combination of the slow resolution of his problems and the data sheet information convinced him that the adhesive was to blame, and he sought some recognition of this. What is perhaps interesting about this case is that the Company involved robustly defended its practices and went to considerable expense and trouble to counter Mr B's claims.

RE: An Expert Report prepared by Dr M.D. Coleman on the instructions of ****
Solicitors concerning the case of Mr B.

Expert qualifications (as in the previous report)

Material instructions

Mr B contends that his exposure to methylene chloride (DCM) in an adhesive known as 'Sta-put' has been responsible for a catalogue of neurological symptoms he has suffered over a period of more than 10 months. I have been requested to comment over whether excessive exposure to DCM could have been responsible for his symptoms.

Dichloromethane and its toxicity

1. In general, non-aromatic solvents such as DCM cause a number of conditions when exposure is chronic. These can include weight loss, anaemia, proteinuria, haematuria and bone marrow hypoplasia [5]. Other symptoms include euphoria, fatigue, anxiety, irritability, headaches, depression, behavioural changes and cognitive disorders [7]. Organic solvents are toxic to skin because they are very effective as de-fatting agents, and this usually leads to dermatitis in most individuals if exposure is high enough.

2. The volatility of the solvents enables them to enter the lungs and become absorbed into the bloodstream within minutes. Solvents can then penetrate the brain within a few minutes, entering the fatty areas of the membranes of the brain cells. Although it is not fully understood how they actually disrupt neural tissue function, they cause a well-defined series of symptoms, which include disorientation, euphoria, ataxia and confusion [5]. DCM is used in a variety of industries, based on its high volatility. It is particularly useful in rapid curing contact adhesives, such as 'Sta-put'. Unfortunately, compared with other organic solvents, DCM has an extra dimension to its toxicity, as it can be converted to carbon monoxide, which reacts with haemoglobin to form carboxyhaemoglobin, which does not carry oxygen. If a modest proportion of blood haemoglobin is converted to carboxyhaemoglobin, this may not markedly affect a healthy individual's ability to work. If the levels rise to 15% and beyond, the effects will start to appear as breathlessness, as well as nausea and fatigue, leading to reduced capacity for work.

3. As the oxygen-carrying capacity is temporarily diminished in this way, the heart must operate at an increased rate to compensate, and *in extremis*, latent heart defects can lead eventually to heart failure. The effects of carboxyhaemoglobin, together with the actions of the parent solvent on the brain, may lead to the CNS symptoms that are usually described for DCM. These include those listed on the data sheet for 'Sta-put', such as light-headedness, depression, fatigue, effects on balance, etc. DCM is also known to exacerbate a number of pre-existing conditions, such as skin, heart, liver and neurological diseases. Mr B's history of heavy

smoking and asthma will have been exacerbated by the effects of DCM on his respiratory system. Mr B's documented experiences involving anger management and anxiety (1996–1997) will presumably be addressed by a separate report from a Neuropsychiatrist and are beyond the remit of this report.

Effects of DCM on Mr B: opportunities for solvent contact

1. The standard for long-term DCM exposure over 8 h is 100 ppm, or 350 mg/m^3. The 15-min exposure is set at 300 ppm, or 1060 mg/m^3. The Company has carried out some tests with the 'Sta-put' product, and they maintain that exposure is less than 20% of the short-term limit. The Company's 'Summary of Results' states that the use of 'Sta-put' is expected to be no more than 10- to 15-s bursts, several times per day. It is not immediately clear from the Company literature whether their tests were carried out in the same room that Mr B worked with the adhesive.

2. With a highly volatile solvent such as DCM, adequate ventilation is essential to avoid exposure to toxic concentrations of the agent. Mr B claims that there was little or no appreciable ventilation in the room where he used the adhesive. In addition, there is a clear disagreement between Mr B's account of the extent of his use of the product and the Company account. This should be possible to partially resolve by accessing Company records on purchase of the adhesive. The usage, in terms of litres of adhesive used, would give some idea as to exposure to the DCM component. Mr B states that the ceilings in the room were 12-ft high.

3. He does not supply any more detail, such as the length of the room, so some estimation of room volume cannot be made. In the absence of adequate ventilation, the degree of exposure Mr B experienced would be directly proportional to the amount of the product he used. Often, organic solvents gradually block the ability to detect them by smell, and Mr B may not have been fully aware of his level of exposure at the time. It would appear likely that the long-term exposure limits for DCM could have been breached on a regular basis in this case.

Evidence of solvent toxicity concerning Mr B

1. Given the degree of exposure that Mr B suggests that he experienced, it would be useful to corroborate this with medical evidence. One measure of Mr B's exposure to DCM would have been the levels of carboxyhaemoglobin in his blood when he was hospitalised. It takes several hours to eliminate all the carboxyhaemoglobin, and since Mr B was exposed to DCM every day, it is possible that levels of carboxyhaemoglobin might accumulate, especially towards the end of a working week. It might be expected that some symptoms resulting from carboxyhaemoglobin, such as breathlessness and a feeling of a lack of fitness, would have been experienced by Mr B.

2. These symptoms are not discussed in his statement. The levels of carboxyhaemoglobin in blood are measured by CO-Oximeters, which are used in hospitals to

measure blood gases. There is some reference to his blood gases being 'unremarkable' in some of the patient notes taken during his admission to hospital (patient notes November 4). In one of the Observation Records for the 3/11, there is a print-out from a Ciba-Corning Blood Gas Analyser. It is apparent from the copy I received that not all of this print-out has been photocopied.

3. However, there is no mention of high carboxyhaemoglobin, and Mr B's blood oxygen saturation is normal. It appears that either carboxyhaemoglobin was not directly measured, or if it was, it was considered within normal limits. The period of hospitalisation from the 3/11 resulted from some neurological disturbances which appear related to those seen in organic solvent toxicity. However, the presence of bacteria in Mr B's blood and his high neutrophil count suggested to the medical staff that he may have been suffering from meningitis. He was given appropriate antibiotic therapy and his symptoms subsided. This episode may well have been unconnected with solvent exposure.

4. The symptoms which disrupted his holiday to Torquay began to improve towards the end of the week, although carboxyhaemoglobin removal from the blood, as well as clearance of the solvent from the brain, should have been complete within hours. This suggests that Mr B's symptoms were more consistent with the clinical profile of those that abuse solvents over long periods of time rather than an acute exposure, where the effects depart in a similar time profile to a 'hangover'. On resumption of his job, Mr B's symptoms also resumed.

Subsequent studies on DCM

1. In 1997, the US Occupational Safety and Health Administration revised its previous long-term limit for DCM from 500 ppm (fivefold higher than that of the United Kingdom) to 25 ppm. This value was decided based on studies on the carcinogenicity of DCM, which is not apparently recognised in the United Kingdom and Europe. The short-term limit was revised down to 125 ppm, which is much less than the 300 ppm the United Kingdom stipulates. The US limits were revised in the face of studies which determined that CNS depression occurs with DCM at levels as low as 175 ppm.

2. Clearly, DCM is believed to be much more toxic in the perception of the United States, compared with that of Europe. It is also apparent, although it is unclear as to whether this is recognised in the United Kingdom, that DCM rapidly penetrates all current air-purifying respirators. The stipulated protection from DCM in the United States is now a complete atmosphere-supply system, where the operators do not breathe any air contaminated with DCM at all. Air compressors and extensive duct work are required to ensure that DCM does not contact the operator in any way [12].

3. The Company could not, of course, be expected to be aware of foreign perceptions of DCM toxicity; however, the agent is capable of causing long-term health damage which is not fully realised in the United Kingdom and Europe. In the light of

the emerging toxicity of DCM and the stringency of US regulations on this agent, it is interesting that Mr B contends that he was only latterly supplied with 'flimsy paper masks', and he also had serious contact with the glue on his body, as well as breathing the fumes.

Summary

1. It is apparent that Mr B's employer did not comply with 'Section 8 Exposure Controls/Personal Protection' as listed in the safety data sheet which accompanied 'Sta-put'. This states that respiratory protection is not required 'if adequate ventilation' is present. Local exhaust is also recommended, as is the provision of impervious gloves. None of these was present. The Company statement even remarked on the effects of the glue on the hands of the operators who performed the exposure tests. It is apparent that the Company did not comply with the safety data sheet recommendations for the period of time that Mr B used the product.

2. Given the frequency of usage of the adhesive, the estimated size of the room and the lack of positive ventilation, it is also probable that the long- and short-term levels of DCM exposure were exceeded when Mr B was using 'Sta-put', although to what degree depends on the exact frequency of his use of the adhesive, which is a matter of dispute. The Company did not appear to be aware of the potential toxicity of DCM and failed in its duty of care to Mr B to adequately protect him from exposure to this solvent. The profile of Mr B's medical symptoms does fit those that would be expected from long-term exposure to DCM. Overall, I believe that the balance of probabilities suggests that Mr B's chronic exposure to excessive concentrations of DCM was responsible for the majority of his health difficulties over the period of March last year to the present day.

M.D. Coleman, Ph.D.,
Lecturer in Toxicology

3.7.1 Case comment

This case was more difficult compared with that of the hexane exposure, in terms of ascribing causality, partly because Mr B had not experienced a catastrophic crisis, but rather, a series of health problems that could have been interpreted quite widely, and indeed Mr B's medical records do reflect a consistent and somewhat fruitless search for 'natural' causes of his problems. Labyrinthitis was considered and then rejected, followed by migraines. The records also comment on the problem of Mr B's anxiety, which was considered as separate from his other symptoms. His attitude to medical examination was also noted to range from being somewhat touchy on some occasions, to actually becoming quite confrontational on others. One report suggested that he might actually be physically dangerous if he acted on his ideas. Such psychological disturbance and aggression could be rooted in any number of personality issues, aside from the intoxicating effects of the solvent. At one point, Mr B was taking up to 14 different medications to combat his problems, ranging from his history of asthma to various possible neurological conditions. Different scans and blood investigations revealed little if anything in the way of a solid cause of his problems.

With hindsight, if an individual is perhaps in effect, repeatedly poisoned, followed by some recovery, in a constant futile cycle by a chemical agent, then it could be argued that it is almost impossible to ascribe causation to any one factor with any certainty, and all medical intervention can become an expensive and gruelling process of 'chasing one's own tail'. In addition, in some cases, the after-effects of the exposure can make the claimant very difficult to deal with due to their instability and irrationality, which can erode sympathy for their dilemma, even amongst professional people used to dealing with the public.

This case was also made more complex by the marked divergence of the Company's account of Mr B's daily exposure to DCM and his own account. The Company criticised my report as being over-reliant on Mr B's testimony, which is a reasonable point, and although I had based my arguments on his medical records and symptoms, if the case had reached court, it may well have hinged on which side made the most convincing argument as to opportunities for exposure to DCM. If the Company could have proved that Mr B spent perhaps only 10 min/day exposed to the glue, then much of the causation reporting would have been redundant, as the 'dose' would have not been sufficient to make a reasonable case for the solvent being responsible for Mr B's symptoms. However, it was clear that Mr B's working environment was generally bereft of effective protective devices of any kind to prevent contact with the glue or the vapour, and it was also apparent that the DCM-laden fumes were liberated in a relatively confined space in the booth which constituted Mr B's workstation. There was no evidence that the Company had given Mr B any guidance as to preventing contamination with the glue, which they should have done, perhaps by the provision of disposable gloves. Interestingly, the case would have been much more accessible to causation attribution had the 'smoking gun' been found, that is, the complete read-out from the CO-Oximeter in the hospital. This might have been expected to show a high level of carboxyhaemo-globin in Mr B's blood – higher than what would have been expected for a modest smoker. Indeed, although CO levels derived from charcoal fires have been esti-mated to be subject to a half-life of around 80 min [13], in the case of CO derived from DCM exposure, the half-life could be as long as 13 h [14]. Hence, it is surprising that the CO level was not recorded. DCM is also viewed as potentially carcinogenic [15], and it is striking that the disparity between the US perception of this solvent and that of Europe has not really changed in the decade or so since this report was written.

3.8   Mr B and dichloromethane: Further developments

After the Company read and digested my original report, they decided to engage another organisation to actually 're-stage' Mr B's daily work activities, by using the adhesive to assemble some furniture units in the booth similar to the one used by Mr B, followed by some *in situ* measurements of DCM concentrations over a brief period of time. These measurements were made by an outside organisation (Organisation X). The DCM concentrations determined in this re-staging exercise were perhaps rather unsurprisingly well below the recommended maximum. The Company insisted that this was a legitimate attempt to explore Mr B's working conditions and that the reported results meant that exposure was in actuality very low and there was thus no case to answer. I was invited by the furniture company's solicitors to write a response to this initiative, and it was made clear that if I did not oblige, then I would be subject to a court order to enforce my compliance. Once you are involved in a case, then you essentially are there to the finish, irrespective of your other commitments. My response was as follows:

*RE: Mr B (d.o.b.****) vs The Manufacturer*

Dear Sir,

In response to your letter of the 13th July

You are asking me to assume that the manufacturer's single-day measurements are typical of those levels experienced by Mr B. As I mentioned in my previous letter, I do not find this assumption credible or plausible. There are too many variables that cannot be reproduced. Irrespective of the defence's ability to prove this in Court, it remains scientifically unacceptable to compare two separate sets of observations derived from vastly different, unknown or disputed conditions.

The NOEL (no observable effect level) of DCM in man was generally assumed to be around 100 ppm, or 347 mg/m³ [16]. The toxicity of DCM has become more apparent as research has progressed, and since 1997, in the United States, 8-h exposure has been set at one-quarter of the 347 mg/m³ value [17]. The levels measured by Organisation X on the day they made their determinations are a fraction even of this value. Nevertheless, Mr B reported symptoms that were strongly consistent with DCM (solvent) toxicity.

A recent study has highlighted the observation that with solvents, CNS toxicity appears to be dependent on the pattern of exposure; the authors state 'that exposure to regularly occurring peak concentrations may have a stronger impact on the brain than constant exposure at the same average level' [18]. Hence, although Organisation X's measurements were carried out assiduously, they measured average levels of DCM over 55–100 min rather than the peak levels, which have the greatest impact on the CNS.

Therefore, scientifically, I feel that Mr B's description of his symptoms is more credible as 'measurement' of contemporaneous DCM concentrations than a single day's retrospective measurements that were unlikely to have borne a close relationship with Mr B's work environment during his employment.

I feel that on the balance of the evidence presented to me, Mr B's symptoms were a result of DCM toxicity.

The long-term toxicity of DCM remains to be fully documented in humans, even though animal studies have shown that the agent is carcinogenic. Regarding any degree of 'organic brain damage', it is very difficult to estimate these things without a full battery of cognitive tests. In the absence a full neurological assessment, it remains my impression that Mr B should have recovered from his exposure, and it is probably not likely that he has sustained permanent injury as a result of his experiences with DCM.

M.D. Coleman, D.Sc.,
Senior Lecturer in Toxicology

3.8.1   Further case comment

The furniture company's legal representation insisted to me in further telephone communications that the issue about the credibility of their 're-staging' exercise was essentially a legal, rather than a scientific one, in that a court might well accept that they had adequately reproduced Mr B's working practices. Hence, because they did not find toxic threshold levels of DCM in the re-staging, then this would support their contention that Mr B was exaggerating his claims of injury and that he was not a credible witness to his own experience. In this case, I felt that it was prudent to maintain the position that the Company's re-staging of the events of 18 months previously without making any attempt to involve the main protagonist, and failing to use the adhesives in the same manner as Mr B was frankly scientifically and legally unconvincing, to put it mildly.

Soon after, I was informed that the Company had settled with Mr B over his health problems. A subsequent Health and Safety investigation did cause the Company to invest more than £20,000 in safety improvements, including the exploration of water-based adhesive alternatives and the restriction on where the DCM adhesive could be used and ventilation improvements were also instigated. The investigation confirmed that Mr B had never received protective gloves or had been supplied with a data sheet detailing the toxicity of DCM when he was handling the adhesive. Whilst the ramifications for the claimant and his family over his working experience were unpleasant and drawn out, the case did lead again to improvement in the working environment for the claimant's former work colleagues, and a medical report also stated that Mr B would make a full recovery.

3.9   Case history 3: Mr C and chronic solvent exposure and behaviour

There is no doubt that breathing high-concentration fumes from aliphatic and aromatic, chlorinated and brominated organic solvents of various types will cause intoxication, followed by CNS depression, unconsciousness and death as outlined earlier. Any tests of concentration, cognition, calculation or other mental activity of an individual exposed to a high level of solvent vapour are likely to parallel those carried out in alcohol-intoxicated individuals. However, as with low-level organophosphate exposure (see Chapter 5, section 12 onwards), what is still hotly debated in the scientific and medical literature is whether chronic occupational organic solvent exposure actually causes structural and functional damage to the human CNS, which can be regarded as a consistent and recognisable syndrome. Furthermore, if this damage occurs, what influence does it have on the individual's behaviour and personality? Since the 1970s, when solvent toxicity was first studied relatively intensively, several terms have emerged which try to describe the chronic occupational effect of organic solvents on the brain; these include 'painter's syndrome', CTE (see Mr A's case) and organic solvent syndrome [19]. Even relatively recent studies have failed to establish whether these syndromes really are a consistent manifestation of solvent exposure [20], despite the application of psychometric tests from the 1980's onwards to those with a working lifetime of solvent exposure, involving cognition and behavioural measurements [21]. The tests can measure whether solvent presence at different concentrations can influence complex tasks, and worker's tolerance can be investigated thoroughly to determine thresholds of solvent presence which affect performance [22]. However, how a history of solvent exposure might influence an individual's response to day-to-day situations in their personal lives is less easily investigated.

Have you ever considered how they make 'tin' cans? The steel ones that contain baked beans, meats and various other foodstuffs? No? Well, since you asked, they start with pieces of rolled mild steel, depending on whether they are making 40 or 80 g cans, which they fold into a cylinder, sealed at one end, which is coated on the inside with a clear lacquer to prevent food contamination. The external seam on the can used to be much larger than it is now, and that was coated with a much thicker 'side-stripe' lacquer to ensure it sealed and did not corrode over the shelf life of the product. The cans are then baked in a huge oven to dry the lacquers, prior to filling with various food products, followed by the sterilisation process and final sealing. So now you are slightly acquainted with some aspects of can making.

The following report describes essentially an attempt at mitigation, as Mr C had committed a serious crime of violence which ended in the death of a woman. They had both worked for several years in a canning factory where the atmosphere was believed to be contaminated on a daily basis with various aromatic and aliphatic solvents. The intention was to determine if the solvent exposure had in some way predisposed Mr C to commit his violent acts. The report was requested to be short and to be produced on a restricted timescale, prior to the criminal trial.

RE: An Expert Report prepared by Dr M.D. Coleman on the instructions of ****
Solicitors concerning the case of Mr C and his occupational solvent exposure.

Material instructions

Mr C is accused of murdering his long-term partner. He worked for a local canning factory from 1974 to 1998, as a fitter in the can-making department. Lacquers and solvents were used in the manufacture of the cans. An opinion is sought as to whether Mr C's exposure to these chemicals, given the fact he was an alcoholic, could have damaged his mental state to the extent that under pressure and provocation and whether he could have reacted in the manner that he did on the day of the killing, some two years and one month after the termination of his employment and the cessation of exposure.

Background

1. Mr C had been in a relationship with his deceased partner for around 14 years, although they did not live together. They met at his employment and worked different shifts in the same area of the factory. By his own admission, his relationship had been 'blissful' for the first 8 years, but deteriorated after that period. It was apparent that Mr C had a number of personal problems, such as his marriage breakdown, his slide into alcoholism followed by dismissal caused by misconduct involving alcohol. In addition, he was epileptic, and his financial affairs appeared to have been chaotic and largely controlled by the deceased.

2. A series of events led to Mr C suspecting that the deceased was appropriating his money and he stated that he wished the relationship to end, but the deceased would not countenance this. In addition, Mr C stated that the deceased had been violent to him on many occasions, including scarring him with a hot iron and threatening him with various sharp implements, such as scissors and knives, which were to hand in the kitchen. Some of the violence had been witnessed by workmates.

3. By the early morning of the victim's death, Mr C had already consumed several prescription drugs, which were termed 'sleeping tablets' by Mr C; in addition, he claimed to have only drunk a single whisky by 08.00 when the victim came to the house he was staying in. A violent argument ensued, where the victim pinned him against the cooker and was verbally abusive. Mr C then asked the victim if she wanted a cup of coffee, and she retired to an adjacent room. Whilst presumably preparing the beverage, he saw a brown handled 6- to 7-in. bread knife and walked into the room and stabbed her. He was pulled away from her by his son and a friend, and he appeared to calm down. He then seized the knife again and stabbed the victim a second time. Following emergency surgery, the victim died 2 h later. His only comment was he was 'sick of her'. When the Police arrived, he admitted that he had stabbed her, but could not account for how many times.

Mr C's working environment

1. Mr C worked as a skilled maintenance fitter in charge of production of cans. After the cans have been produced, they were coated with side-stripe lacquer, which contained several organic solvents. The cans were initially cleaned with a degreasant, identified by Mr C as 'Genklene™', which is a trade name for 1,1,1-trichloroethane (methyl chloroform). After 1987, Mr C recorded that the Company abruptly stopped using this agent. He described in his statement how he was constantly 'getting covered' in the lacquer and the Genklene. The cans were then baked after being rolled and he remarked that this generated a great deal of fumes. Mr C mentioned that many people in the canning shop were affected by these fumes, and another letter from a colleague of Mr C stated that many of the ladies who worked in this area were quite badly affected, despite the Company's attempts to improve ventilation. One lady had resigned due to ill-health and she had spent 20 years working in the same environment. This lady claimed that her colleagues all had chest and throat problems, and at least one other person had tried to take the Company to court over their health problems, but no claim was successful.

Types of solvents used in the Company

1. The 1,1,1-trichloroethane in Genklene™ has a considerable literature regarding its toxicity to man, including damage to the kidneys, liver and brain [23, 24] and is also thought to be carcinogenic [25]. At least two variants of lacquer were employed, one for the internal coating of the cans to prevent metal contamination of the food and the other (side stripe) to seal the external can joint after it has been rolled into shape.

2. Both lacquers contained amino and epoxy resin mixtures, which were carried by several solvents, including methyl ethyl ketone, (25%) toluene (10–25%), xylene (10%), 2-butoxyethanol (10–25%) and ethyl acetate (25–50%). It is likely that the majority of the workers' exposure to these solvents would have been by inhalation, as well as a minor component through skin absorption [26].

3. Studies conducted on workers in Japan exposed to combinations of solvents similar to those mentioned earlier, containing ethyl acetate, methyl isobutylketone and toluene, reported CNS depression and local irritation, although the authors considered that there were no metabolic interactions between the solvents. There was no indication that the toxicity of toluene was modified by concurrent exposure to the other agents [27]. However, many studies have underlined the cumulative effects of solvent toxicity on the CNS, which may lead to 'CTE'. Effects on the human brain include damage to memory, ability to concentrate, awareness and the tendency to general mood swings and long-term psychological depression.

4. The most commonly implicated solvents in this type of toxicity include xylene and toluene as well as 1,1,1-trichloroethane [19, 28]. I think it is clear that the Company should have been aware that solvent hazes and mists are toxic, and specifically, they are neurotoxic, so are likely to pose a threat to Plant Safety as well as to the

individual concerned. The toxicity of various organic solvents has been common knowledge in industry for more than 25 years, and the Company would be reasonably expected to have been aware of the potential danger of these hazards.

Epilepsy and solvent exposure

1. Mr C suffered from epilepsy and there is relatively little evidence on how solvent exposure affects this condition. Whilst acute solvent exposure can cause convulsions [29], in the opinion of some experts, solvent exposure may make existing epileptic conditions worse [30]. There is some evidence that exposure to various pollutant chemicals, such as those encountered in the workplace, can affect experimental animal and probably human sensitivity to several CNS disorders and exacerbate them. These can range from behavioural problems such as panic attacks [31] to other more complex conditions such as epilepsy [32]. The effects of solvent exposure on liver metabolising enzymes may also impact the clearance and therefore the pharmacological action of anti-epileptic drugs [28].

Effects of alcohol abuse and solvent exposure

1. Mr C suffered from alcoholism and this impacted his life to the extent that he ultimately lost his job through his poor time-keeping and performance, despite the Company making efforts to support him during his condition, as evidenced by contact between Mr C's General Practitioner and the Company. He did receive a payoff from the Company after an enquiry conducted by an Industrial Tribunal. There is evidence that alcohol acts in a similar manner to other solvents in its impact on the CNS, and it is likely at least to have an additive effect on the potential neurotoxic action of solvents [33].

2. Regarding exposure to the specific solvents, Mr C worked in an atmosphere which contained toluene, which is metabolised to hippuric acid by the same enzyme systems which metabolizes ethanol; this in effect means that when an individual has consumed large amounts of ethanol, their alcohol intake acts to inhibit the enzymes which remove toluene, and the solvent can accumulate in the individual's body and CNS, making its neurotoxicity worse [34].

3. There is also evidence that other solvents related to toluene, such as xylene, as well as several ketones are also metabolised by the same enzyme systems as ethanol; some studies have indicated that the effects are non-linear and thus are very difficult to predict, but nonetheless show that the CNS effects of these solvents are increased by ethanol usage [35]. Hence, there is a strong probability that Mr C's alcohol intake will have caused any solvent-related CNS effects to exert a more potent toxic impact on his behaviour, as well as his cognitive and reasoning powers.

Opinion

The scientific literature suggests strongly that Mr C's solvent exposure and alcohol consumption may have affected his behaviour during his work at the Company.

However, given the lack of conclusive evidence in the scientific literature for the existence of occupationally related solvent encephalopathies (such as CTE), it is much harder to predict whether these problems, in terms of impact on cognition, reasoning and behaviour, would have persisted for the period of time which encompassed the killing of Mr C's partner. It could be suggested that Mr C should undergo a battery of neuro-cognitive and behavioural tests which might explore the degree of deterioration he may have suffered in comparison with what should be expected as 'normal' for his age. The outcome of these tests might then provide some context for mitigation for the offence he committed.

M.D. Coleman,
Lecturer in Toxicology

3.9.1   Case comment

The documentation of this case was complex and often contradictory. A letter was included that was written by a factory worker, which stated that the ladies who worked in the can fabrication section were 'do-lally' because of the solvents. Certainly, the Company submitted documentation, which showed that it was aware of cases where workers had complained about solvent fumes and letters were available from the spouses of women who they felt had suffered severely from their employment with the Company. To be fair, at least one spouse of a sufferer did report that their extensive contact with Occupational Health personnel within the Company met with care and consideration. One letter mentioned the presence of 'blue grey fumes' from the baking of the lacquers onto the cans, and it was stated that none of the workers was ever given any information on the hazards related to the solvents and fumes to which they were exposed. In my examination of the supplied documentation, I could see how the Company responded to a written complaint. Their letter employed a rather incongruous mixture of sympathy, reasonable supporting evidence and unambiguous legal threats to sue if 'false or malicious allegations' were to be made in public. Another letter from the husband of a worker stated that ventilation had recently been restricted, whilst the Company stated that they had actually passed Health and Safety Executive and other external inspections without any problems. The cause of the spouse of an individual who had been retired due to ill-health was perhaps somewhat hamstrung by the Company allowing his wife's retirement on a medical condition which was not related to solvent effects, although he was adamant that her health had improved immeasurably since she had left her occupation. To the external observer, the documentation suggests that the working environment at the factory was not optimal in terms of the solvent fumes and it is also highly likely that these fumes did impact the workers' lives.

Since solvents are known for their tendency to cause behavioural changes which can be manifested in mood changes, irrationality, irritability, panic attacks and other signs of mental instability, Mr C and his partner's already volatile relationship would have almost certainly been made significantly worse by their shared place of work. It is a matter for conjecture as to how much of the victim's difficult behaviour, such as her instability and aggression toward the defendant, might be in part linked to her own exposure to the solvents. Indeed, documentation was supplied describing attempts made 2 years previously by third parties to formulate a case for compensation for Mr C after he was dismissed from the Company. This letter pointed out that attempts were largely thwarted by the sheer irrationality of Mr C's partner, even though paradoxically she was trying to support Mr C to the best of her ability. That the victim's behaviour was influenced by the solvents was also the opinion of the spouse of the lady that had to retire due to ill-health. However, these are all just opinions, and it will never be known how much the victim herself was damaged by her work.

Mr C's defence team took up the suggestion made in my report that he should undergo the battery of tests of competence, general cognitive and behavioural assessment, although unfortunately for him, he did rather too well. Despite his history of alcohol abuse and solvent exposure, he tested as normal, so he could not claim mitigation for his act on the basis of the solvent exposure, and he was convicted of manslaughter. In effect, Mr C was judged to have recovered from his solvent exposure and was fully responsible for his actions. In hindsight, it is tempting to speculate how events might have unfolded had the two protagonists worked in a different environment.

3.10 Summary of chronic solvent toxicity and behaviour

These reports demonstrate some of the complexity of individual cases and the significant conflicts in the respective perceptions of the claimants and the defendants. Whilst the first case demonstrates that a severe and life-threatening experience at first glance looks certain to be linked with occupation, a case must still be made to rule out other factors which could possibly exert influence. The second and third histories underline the idea of conflicts in evidence with regard to exposure – all the most detailed and persuasive causation cellular mechanism–based explanations are worthless if the claimant cannot provide enough evidence that they received a sufficient 'toxic dose' to cause their problems. Also in the latter two cases, the employer could argue that they had complied with all external strictures and inspections and that the dose could not have been as high as the worker's symptoms suggest. Somewhat ironically, the final history also underlines the remarkable toughness of the human brain, where it can withstand significant chemical 'punishment' over many years from a variety of sources, apparently without measurable lasting impact on its cognitive powers.

References

1. Harris MO, Corcoran J, Agency for Toxic Substances and Disease Registry. Toxicological Profile for *n*-Hexane. U.S. Department of Health and Human Services, Public Health Service, Atlanta, 1–230, 1999.
2. Sendur OF et al. Toxic neuropathy due to N-hexane: report of three cases. Inhal Toxicol. 21, 210–214, 2009.
3. Woehrling EK, Zilz TR, Coleman MD. The effects of hexanediones on neural and astrocytic cell lines. Env Tox Pharmacol. 22, 249–254, 2006.
4. Chan R. Chinese Workers Appeal to Apple Over Health Worries. Reuters.com, http://uk.reuters.com/article/2011/02/22/oukin-uk-apple-wintek-idUKTRE71L22520110222 (accessed on 22 February 2011).
5. Stacy NH. Toxicity of organic solvents. In: Occupational Toxicology. Taylor & Francis, London, 205–213, 1995.
6. Collings AJ, Luxton SG, editors. The Safe Use of Solvents. Academic Press, New York, 1982.
7. Tahti H et al. Organic solvents. In: Ballantyne B et al., editors. General and Applied Toxicology, 2nd edition. Macmillan, Oxford, 2028–2047, 1998.
8. Okudaira K et al. Inhalant abusers and psychiatric symptoms. Seishin Shinkeigaku Zasshi. 98, 203–212, 1996.
9. Saito T. Clinical manifestation of volatile solvent psychosis (English Abstract). NAYIZ. 32, 189–196, 1997.
10. Mikkelsen S. Epidemiological update on solvent neurotoxicity. Environ Res. 73, 101–112, 1997.
11. Ng TP et al. Neurobehavioral effects of industrial mixed solvent exposure in Chinese printing and paint workers. Neurotoxicol Teratol. 12, 661–664, 1990.
12. Methylene Chloride; Final Rule OSHA, Department of Labor, www.osha.gov (accessed on 11 November 13).
13. Li CK. A retrospective study on carboxyhaemoglobin half-life in acute carbon monoxide poisoning in patients treated with normobaric high flow oxygen. Hong Kong J Emerg Med. 13, 205–211, 2006.
14. Dichloromethane: Human Health Effects Toxnet. http://toxnet.nlm.nih.gov/cgi-bin/sis/search/a?dbs+hsdb:@term+@DOCNO+66 (accessed on 11 November 13).
15. DHHS/National Toxicology Program; Eleventh Report on Carcinogens: Dichloromethane (75-09-2) http://ntp.niehs.nih.gov/ntp/roc/eleventh/profiles/s066dich.pdf (accessed on 11 November 2013).
16. Ott MG et al. Health evaluation of employees exposed to methylene chloride. Metabolism data and oxygen half-saturation pressures. Scand J Work Environ Health. 9(Suppl 1), 31–38, 1983.
17. Fan A, Alexeeff GV. Public Health Goal for Dichloromethane: Dichloromethane (Methylene Chloride, DCM). Office of Environmental Health Hazard Assessment, Sacramento, 1–137, 2000.
18. Lammers JHCM et al. Neurobehavioural evaluation and kinetics of inhalation of constant or fluctuating toluene concentrations in human volunteers. Environ Toxicol Pharmacol. 20, 431–442, 2005.
19. Ridgway TE et al. Occupational exposure to organic solvents and long-term nervous system damage detectable by brain imaging, neurophysiology or histopathology. Food Chem Toxicol. 41, 153–187, 2003.

20. Matsuoka M. Neurotoxicity of organic solvents – recent findings. Brain Nerve. 59, 591–596, 2007.
21. Gamberale F. Use of behavioural performance tests in the assessment of solvent toxicity. Scand J Work Environ Health. 1(Suppl 1), 65–74, 1985.
22. van Thriel C et al. From neurotoxic to chemosensory effects: new insights on acute solvent neurotoxicity exemplified by acute effects of 2-ethylhexanol. Neurotoxicology. 28, 347–355, 2007.
23. Cohen C, Frank AL. Liver disease following occupational exposure to 1,1,1-trichloroethane: a case report. Am J Ind Med. 26, 237–241, 1994.
24. Flanagan RJ, Ives R. Volatile substance abuse. Bull Narc. 46, 49–78, 1994.
25. Anttila A et al. Cancer incidence among Finnish workers exposed to halogenated hydrocarbons. J Occup Environ Med. 37, 797–806, 1995.
26. Kezic S et al. Skin absorption of some solvent vapours in volunteers. Int Arch Occup Environ Health. 73, 415–422, 2000.
27. Ukai H et al. Occupational exposure of solvent mixtures-effects on health and metabolism. Occup Environ Med. 51, 523–529, 1994.
28. Viaene MK. Overview of the neurotoxic effects in solvent-exposed workers. Arch Public Health. 60, 217–232, 2002.
29. Pryor GT. Solvent-induced neurotoxicity: effects and mechanisms. In: Chang LW, Dyer RS, editors. Handbook of Neurotoxicology. Marcel Dekker, Inc., New York, 377–400, 1995.
30. White R. Clinical neuropathological investigation of solvent neurotoxicity. In: Chang LW, Dyer RS, editors. Handbook of Neurotoxicology. Marcel Dekker, Inc., New York, 335–376, 1995.
31. Dager SR et al. Panic disorder precipitated by exposure to organic solvents in the workplace. Am J Psychiatry. 144, 1056–1058, 1987.
32. Bell IR et al. Testing the neural sensitization and kindling hypothesis for illness from low levels of environmental chemicals. Environ Health Perspect. 105(Suppl 2), 539–547, 1997.
33. Cherry NM et al. Organic brain damage and occupational solvent exposure. Br J Ind Med. 49, 776–781, 1992.
34. Baelum J. Human solvent exposure-factors influencing the pharmacokinetics and acute toxicity. Pharmacol Toxicol. 68(Suppl 1), 1–36, 1991.
35. MacDonald AJ et al. Analysis of solvent central nervous system toxicity and ethanol interactions using a human population physiologically based kinetic and dynamic model. Regul Toxicol Pharmacol. 35, 165–176, 2002.

4
Chronic and permanent injury: Bladder cancer and occupation

4.1 Bladder cancer

According to Cancer Research UK's figures for 2010, bladder cancer was the fourth most common cancer reported in males, with 7416 individuals affected, which is 4.5% of all cases recorded that year [1]. The disease is much less common in females, so overall, it is the seventh commonest cancer, with over 10,000 new cases in 2010. Five-year survival has steadily improved since I started writing causation reports in this area; I recall survivals for males which were around 35% in 1997, which have risen to over 71% currently [1], although it is 10% lower for women. However, the main treatment still involves surgery and/or radiotherapy and chemotherapy. Whilst it is often difficult to directly ascribe a cause to a specific cancer, the strongest risk for developing this disease is to be male and to smoke. In Chapter 1, the carcinogenic potential of polycyclic aromatic hydrocarbons (PAHs) was discussed at length, and a sub-group of these agents, the aromatic amines, are responsible for bladder cancer in smokers as well as in neoplasms of occupational origin.

Aromatic amines were used as antioxidants in a variety of industries, particularly in rubber, printing and dye manufacture, but the relatively early realisation in the twentieth century that they were specifically carcinogens of the bladder led to their removal from most processes. This means that unless a working career started in the 1940s and 1950s, it is difficult to prove that an individual was specifically exposed to aromatic amines. However, there remains to this day (after adjustment for smoking history) a strong occupational risk factor for the development of bladder cancer in men, which is not present for women [2], which means that if a male works in one of the 'usual suspect' industries, such as petrochemicals, cars, dyes, tyres or light engineering, they are either still being exposed to aromatic amines, which are perhaps now being formed inadvertently during manufacturing processes, or they are other previously unsuspected agents which are also potent bladder carcinogens, or a combination of both factors. Either way, it is clear that occupational

Expert Report Writing in Toxicology: Forensic, Scientific and Legal Aspects,
First Edition. Michael D. Coleman.
© 2014 John Wiley & Sons, Ltd. Published 2014 by John Wiley & Sons, Ltd.

bladder cancer has not disappeared into the past, and in the future, causation reports will have to find agents which are, on the balance of probabilities, responsible for the condition.

My own involvement with causation report writing began with this type of case, as I had worked for several years on the toxicity of a drug called dapsone, which is an aromatic amine, and I had made a study on the mechanisms of its toxicity as well as strategies to ameliorate some of them [3].

4.2   The patient's perspective

Bladder cancer, like all cancers, makes huge changes in the life of the victim. The initial signs are usually blood in the urine, and investigation might lead to a diagnosis of the stage of the disease. The system used to clinically describe bladder cancers is similar to other cancers, in that it describes where the tumour mass is, whether it has spread to the lymph nodes and finally whether it has metastasised to the rest of the body. This is termed TNM staging:

> T (tumour) can be followed by four numbers as well as letters, which describe how far the tumour mass has developed, in terms of whether it has just appeared as a recognisable tumour, called Ta (non-invasive) all the way to T4, where it has broken out of the bladder and invaded adjacent organs and tissues.
>
> N (nodes) describes whether the tumour has reached local lymph nodes in the vicinity of the tumour and is designated according to the number of local nodes involved, such as N3 for three nodes along the iliac artery.
>
> M (metastasis) a designation of M0 means that the tumour is contained within the bladder, whereas M1 means that it has escaped the bladder.

The information given earlier is combined to provide a stage diagnosis, ranging from stage 0 (no escape or spread) to stage IV, where it has reached other organs and lymph nodes. The grade or general vigour of the cells is also considered. Once a diagnosis has been reached, either surgical, radiotherapeutic or chemotherapeutic options are pursued, either singly or in combination. Surgery can involve the removal of the bladder and other adjacent organs, which makes radical changes to an individual's day-to-day experience. In males, the prostate may also be removed, resulting in loss of fertility, and if the nerves are damaged during surgery, loss of sexual performance too. Although a substitute bladder can be fashioned out of parts of the bowel, the patient may well be left with an external hole or stoma, where the urine drains out into a bag [4, 5]. There are many issues for the patient to confront, not least the changes to their body and the practical aspects of life that they now face, as well as the psychological impact of such a change, which is particularly hard to confront for male patients. For this situation to arise as a result of a somewhat arbitrary decision as a 16- to 18-year-old as to which job advertisement to answer must be extremely difficult to rationalise.

4.3   Bladder cancer: Causes and risks

As outlined in Chapter 1, bladder cancer is strongly associated with aromatic amines, particularly those involved in the dye and rubber industries, namely 4-aminobiphenyl and β-naphthylamine (BNA). The latter compound is also present in tobacco smoke, and it is responsible for bladder cancer linked to tobacco usage [6]. Aromatic amines such as BNA are so dangerous, not because of what they are *per se*, but because of how human metabolising systems change them chemically to clear them from the body. Essentially, a fat-soluble potential toxin such as BNA would not leave the body unless it was made into a water-soluble form which the kidneys could excrete. So the liver, gut and to some extent the kidney and the lung can metabolise aromatic amines by changing their amine groups into hydroxy-lamines. This latter structure is very slightly water soluble and more reactive, so therefore amenable to a second stage of metabolism, where a modified form of glucose is attached to the hydroxylamine to make a glucuronide [7]. This latter metabolite is very water soluble so it can be removed from the blood by the kidney followed by concentration in the urine. However, glucuronides of aromatic amines and to a lesser extent, those of PAHs, are not very stable in urine in the bladder due to the presence of various enzymes and the glucuronides disintegrate, forming reactive metabolites. This is unfortunately a situation rather like a hand grenade with the pin pulled out; these metabolites, such as positively charged nitrenium ions (Figure 4.1) attack the predominantly negatively charged DNA [7]. Over many years, a battle is fought, where the metabolites damage the bladder DNA, and the bladder repairs the damage. At some point, irreversible changes to specific genes occur which are retained in the cellular genome, eventually leading to a malignancy. Clearly, every person who worked in the rubber industry does not develop cancer, so the process is much more complex than is fully understood. There are myriad genetic factors and enzyme systems that protect an individual and others that make them more vulnerable. These factors, such as acetylation status, have been exten-sively investigated [2], and they are beyond the scope of this book and they are also irrelevant as far as ascribing causation in a written report. This is because the sus-ceptibility of the individual is something that they have no power over or knowledge of, so there is no benefit in mentioning it in a report. The technology exists today to genetically assess individuals as to whether they have genes which confer vulnera-bility to certain toxins, and it could be suggested that perhaps this information could be used to prevent recruitment of future victims of such toxins. However, this is no substitute for making the workplace safe and exposure to carcinogens negligible, as there are limits to our knowledge in these areas.

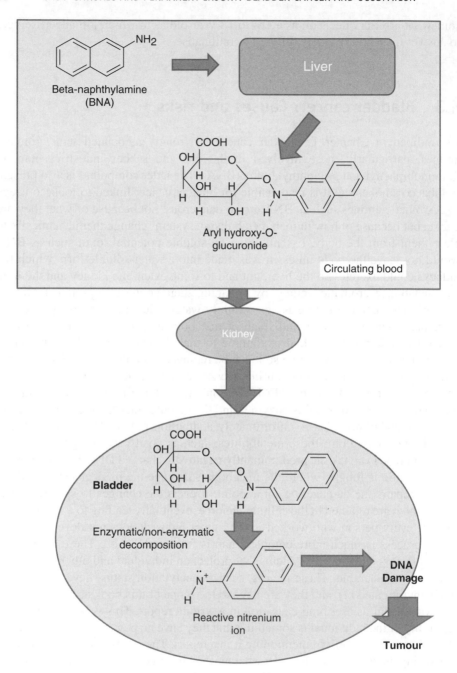

Figure 4.1 Carcinogens such as BNA enter the body and are metabolised to more water-soluble glucuronide products which can be cleared by the kidneys. Unfortunately, these glucuronides decompose in the bladder, creating toxic species such as nitrenium ions, which attack DNA, leading sometimes many decades later to a bladder tumour

4.4   Bladder cancer and occupation: Industrial injury benefit claims

As mentioned in Chapter 2, beginning the process of claiming industrial injury disablement benefit is the first major step an individual might make to gain financial support to ease their day-to-day lives. This is often the only course of redress available to those who might be unable to mount any legal case, either for health or financial reasons, or because there is in effect no single 'target' to sue which possesses the wealth capable of making the claim good financially. Many companies or organisations go out of business or are absorbed by other organisations, which may or may not acknowledge any historic liabilities related to the former entity. In some cases, an entire sector of industry ceases to exist, as with the British-owned and managed car industry. So many individuals might have worked for several companies which have long since passed into history and are in effect beyond legal retribution. An industrial injury benefit claim is their only hope for financial assistance to supplement any existing benefits and/or pensions.

Claims which involve aromatic amine exposure contain several common threads; firstly, they involve latency periods which can exceed 30 years before a neoplasm results. Secondly, from a legal perspective, very few chemicals are recognised by the Department of Work and Pensions (DWP) as *bona fide* causes of bladder cancer, and these are listed in Chapter 2 in Section 2.2. As mentioned in Chapter 2, if an individual is suffering from bladder cancer and they wish to claim benefits, the onus is on them to provide evidence that they were exposed to the prescribed aromatic amines which were, of course, banned decades previously.

It is not easy to prove that a bladder cancer has been linked to occupation to the satisfaction of the DWP and the following cases involved assisting individuals who had developed the disease and had been treated, or were undergoing treatment and had then tried unsuccessfully to claim disability benefit. I either submitted a letter of support, or in some cases, I was permitted to attend their appeal hearings. In some instances, the claimants did win a successful re-examination of their case, but in another case, it was not successful. The process varies slightly from area to area, and the appeal tribunal might consist of a chairman and a medical practitioner or even two practitioners.

4.5   Case history 1: Mr D

This case involved a gentleman who had started his working life in the late 1940s and worked until 1989 as a machinist for many different engineering companies. He supplied me with a brief oral history of his daily work experience, which involved using a variety of different lathes, which bored, cut and shaped steel components of machine tools which were usually used in the car industry. During his career, he was exposed to a wide variety of different unrefined mineral oils which contained high aromatic contents, as well as different oil emulsions which contained amine-based antioxidants. He developed bladder cancer in 1988 and was forced to retire due to ill-health. I wrote the following letter in support of his claim for an industrial injury disablement benefit.

The Benefits Agency,
(Industrial Injuries)

To whom it may concern,

I am writing in support of Mr D's claim for Industrial Injury Disablement Benefit. Mr D was employed as a machinist from 1949 to 1989, where he was exposed to a variety of cutting oils which were used to cool metals during the machining process. These oils fell into a number of categories: neat oils, which until the late 1970s contained many carcinogenic aromatic hydrocarbons and aromatic amines; oil/water mixes, or suds, which contained a fraction of neat oil plus water and several antioxidants and finishing agents; synthetic oils which contained ethanolamine antioxidants and, finally, synthetic oils which contained no dangerous additives. The neat oils would have contained anything up to 20% aromatic hydrocarbons, which are carcinogenic, and some contained antioxidants such as BNA. It is established that 1949 was the final year of manufacture of BNA in the United Kingdom, so it is unlikely to have been present in oils much beyond the early 1950s, although as an impurity in certain neat oils, BNA was present up to the late 1960s. After 1949, there is evidence in the rubber and dye industries that stocks of BNA held by various manufactures were still used up to 2 years after the manufacture ceased. As there has always been a need for the incorporation of antioxidants in cutting oil formulation, it is highly likely that for a relatively short time, from 1949 to the early 1950s, Mr D will have been exposed to BNA in some of the products he was using. It has been documented by various engineering and automotive firms that their cutting oils underwent considerable recycling to cut costs, which, alongside heat-mediated catalytic cracking processes, would increase the concentrations of carcinogenic substances such as BNA. The general levels of personal contamination with oil in the 1940s through to the 1970s would not be tolerated today. Usually, workers operated in very hot environments, with few opportunities for rehydration. Consequently, their urine would have been much more concentrated than is desirable, and the carcinogenic derivatives of BNA would have been present in higher concentrations in these individuals compared with those who were adequately hydrated. BNA is a very potent human bladder carcinogen and only requires minimal exposure to set in motion the long-term cellular changes that eventually lead to bladder cancer. Even less than 2 years of exposure would have been enough to cause Mr D's condition. Long lag-times between exposure to the bladder carcinogen and the appearance of the cancer itself are not unusual. Periods of greater than 40 years have been documented. As a non-smoker, it is not likely that Mr D was exposed to other sources of BNA, such as cigarette smoke. Statistically, the primary cause of bladder cancer is smoking, although it is only the 11th most common cancer and is relatively rare. It is not that common in smokers, as they are more than nine times more likely to develop lung cancer than bladder cancer. Non-smokers do develop bladder cancer, sometimes due to genetic influences, although it is exceedingly rare for this to occur. However, nobody in Mr D's family to his knowledge has developed the disease, and I believe that the balance of probabilities indicates that Mr D's occupation caused his condition and that he worked in an environment where BNA was handled and liberated, and this chemical was the causative agent of his cancer.

Yours faithfully,
Dr M.D. Coleman,
Lecturer in Toxicology

The local benefits agency asked for further clarification with regard to the agents to which Mr D was/may have been exposed:

Dear Ms X

I must apologise for my tardiness in replying to your letter of the 12th of Feb; unfortunately, I have been rather ill, and I am only now catching up with things.

Regarding Mr D, I can confirm that the BNA mentioned in my letter is listed as a C23 category agent; it is in your list at a, (i) after alpha-naphthylamine. This agent is one of the few internationally recognised as a carcinogen of a specific organ. As I stated in my support letter, BNA was used in a number of oil products, although it was replaced in the 1950s by other agents such as PBNA, or phenyl-beta naphthylamine, which is closely related chemically to BNA. This agent could be described as is listed at a, (ii) 'diphenyl substituted', and it is metabolised to BNA in humans and animals. This is also carcinogenic in man.

If you require any more information, please contact me, either by post or email at m.d.coleman@aston.ac.uk

Best Wishes,
Dr M.D. Coleman

A short time later, Mr D was advised that his claim had been successful. This was a very fair judgement, as he would have had no chance at all in obtaining any legal redress, as he had worked for so many commercial concerns over the years and most of them no longer existed. He had been through surgery to remove his bladder and his quality of life was poor, so the pension made a significant difference to his day-to-day expenses. As this was essentially a non-judicial hearing, the benefits agency allowed me to make an argument without extensive referencing to support my statements. It is possible that in future submissions, they might require such detail, which would not be unreasonable.

4.6   Case history 2: Mr E

I have to confess to an abiding and intense love of very large, fast and thirsty cars and how they work, and I also secretly love repairing pretty much any car. However, until I became involved with these cases, I did not give much thought as to who actually made cars and what their working conditions were like.

Mr E worked for 35 years for a car manufacturer in their main body plant. As you are probably aware, car building is a combination of manufacturing, where parts are machined, stamped, pressed, milled and ground, then assembly, to make the finished car. Cars were first built around a basic chassis or framework which was like a steel ladder laid out flat, with the wheels and running gear attached. The car body, which was often made elsewhere, was then bolted to the chassis. Some four-wheel drive vehicles are still made this way, as are truck trailers. This system is very rigid and exceptionally strong, but heavy and not fuel efficient. For decades, passenger cars and now most four-wheel drive off-roaders have been made in a unitary way, where they don't actually have a chassis, but rather a system of box sections welded together complete with a floor and a roof, which all act to provide strength and rigidity to the structure. Convertibles (or dropheads, in correct UK terminology) are more expensive to buy and are a bit slower than the parent car, because they are built with a roof which is then cut off and the underneath sections are strengthened, which makes them heavier. An ex-Ford car worker I knew in Huyton, near Liverpool, used essentially the same process to produce possibly the only Mk.3 Vauxhall Viva convertible that ever existed. Working in the open air outside his house, Kevin also designed and fabricated a folding roof, and the whole structure was declared road legal by his local Ministry of Transport Testing Station.

The previous section was a rather gratuitous way to arrive at telling you that modern cars are built from many sections which have to be prefabricated by pressing or stamping in mild steel, which is very prone to rusting. You only have to look at your car brake discs which are made of cast iron, which rust within a few hours of your last trip. Modern car box sections are galvanised using zinc to prevent rusting, but up to the 1980s, manufacturers used to prevent corrosion by coating all components in very light oils, which would prevent rust, but it would mean that when the box sections were welded together, the welding process would create considerable amounts of fumes from the burning oils, which would liberate carcinogenic aromatic hydrocarbons. The oils themselves would have to be sprayed rather wastefully onto the cars, and they were not very highly refined, so they already contained many aromatic hydrocarbons. Mr E worked as a maintenance fitter on the assembly lines, and his main duties involved working in or around the welding processing of the sections, and he was exposed through inhalation to a combination of oil mist and combustion haze during the welding process. He also had to work at close quarters with the line machinery, crawling through confined and oily spaces. This led to a great deal of physical contamination with the oil, throughout Mr E's working life. He developed bladder cancer at the age of 62, and his condition deteriorated significantly by the time I went with him to the appeal of his case.

The tribunal had originally rejected his case on the basis that he could not prove that he had been exposed to the aromatic amines listed in section C23, which is actually not unreasonable in the context of the Department of Health's guidelines. I made a verbal argument that it was likely that during the combustion process, various aromatic amines would have been formed and that he would have been exposed to chemicals listed in sections C23, as many of the poorly refined oils used at the time he was working contained high levels of aromatics and were used throughout the car industry from the early 1960s. The appeal tribunal accepted my argument, and Mr E was awarded a pension. Three months after I gave him a lift home from the hearing, he died as a result of his condition.

4.7   Case history 3: Mr F

Mr F (born 1926) worked for a large tyre manufacturer as a 'millman' from 1959 to 1986, and he developed bladder cancer in his late 60s. He had been engaged in the manipulation and cutting of processed rubber blocks, prior to their moulding into tyre carcasses. Tyres are made from a combination of synthetic rubber (styrene–butadiene copolymer) and natural rubber, as well as various additive antioxidants and agents to alter the hardness or softness of the tyre according to different performance requirements. As described previously, prior to 1949, BNA was an effective antioxidant which retarded tyre deterioration, but was banned in the United Kingdom. However, it was manufactured and incorporated into rubber products until the early 1970s in countries outside the United Kingdom. It was common knowledge in the rubber industry that many types of tyre, including those manufactured abroad, were recycled by the various manufacturers around the United Kingdom and used to make new tyres, so it was possible that up to the early 1970s, an individual could have been exposed to BNA, and given the long latency of bladder cancer, it was plausible that it could have been implicated as the cause of Mr F's malignancy. Mr F died in 2000 as a result of his condition, and his family sought to gain recognition that his death was caused by his occupation.

Their first submission was refused on the grounds that his employers stated that they had ceased to use BNA in 1949 and that other experts had reported that nobody who worked in the industry after 1951 would be at risk from BNA. In an appeal, it was suggested that Mr F could have been exposed to C23-type agents from the recycling of foreign tyres and rubber sourced from outside the United Kingdom. The tribunal requested from the owners of the factory as to whether they had engaged in this practice, and the Company Doctor sent an emphatically negative reply – that the Company only used its own recycled rubber in its operations. At this point, the tribunal refused the application with the statement that the claimant had 'not discharged the onus of proof' that he had handled C23 listed agents.

In retrospect, it strains credulity that the Company somehow arranged for all recycled rubber to be only their own tyres or that they might have meticulously separated all the recycled rubber into piles, with one perhaps marked 'UK origin' and the other 'from somewhere else and therefore to be sent to landfill'. Recycling operations are often somewhat marginal in their financial viability, and any added expense in sorting rubber according to origin would certainly render the recycling process uneconomic.

If this case had reached a court, it probably would have hinged on whether the claimant could prove that the Company had recycled foreign tyres, which would have meant gathering a great deal of eye-witness testimony of those that were engaged in the recycling operation at the time. Assuming the presence of the foreign tyres was established, causation would have probably have focussed on whether the amounts of BNA involved could plausibly had been enough to cause malignancy.

Of course, it was clearly not in the Company's financial interest to agree that Mr F was harmed by his employment, as it might open the door to litigation from other sufferers. However, one wonders if the decision on behalf of the benefits agency might have been different if Mr F had not died in 2000 and had been able to represent himself, thus demonstrating his direct need for the financial support to improve his quality of life.

4.8 Case history 4: Mrs G

Mrs G worked for a tyre and rubber processing plant, but she was an administrator who carried out her duties in an office above the main manufacturing area. She had held this position for more than 30 years and, in her late 50s, developed bladder cancer. Mrs G's initial application for disability benefit was turned down, probably because she worked in the office, she could not demonstrate in her application that she had been in sufficient contact with synthetic rubber-related material. However, on appeal, I accompanied her to the tribunal, and I made the point that as a woman and a non-smoker, the odds of her developing bladder cancer with no disease family history would normally be very remote. The crucial evidence was a remark she made about her duties first thing in the morning; she opened the office door, and she always had to find a small brush and remove the fine black dust which had settled on every surface in the room. She was asked to provide a map of where the office was in relation to the production facility, and it became obvious that she had been breathing processed rubber dust for her whole working life. Since she had worked in the factory before the 1970s, it was possible that she had been exposed to BNA in any recycled rubber that might have been used in the factory. Hence, the tribunal found in her favour, despite a lack of precision in her exposure attribution in terms of section C23.

4.9   Bladder cancer and occupation: Legal claims for compensation

As described in chapter 2.2, earlier, if an individual successfully makes a claim for Industrial Injuries Disablement Benefit, this can assist in day-to-day issues such as the costs of materials which support their condition. However, a claim for disability might be denied to someone else, for example, on the basis that the claimant could not prove that a C23 agent caused their bladder cancer. Both individuals would still require some redress, primarily based on a public recognition of who is responsible for their condition, as well as some financial compensation. This is most likely to be sought through a legal claim for damages. Of course, it is worth stating that if the claimant's former employers are still trading or functioning, then a successful disability pension claim does not preclude making an approach for compensation. In the following two cases, there was a clear target: in the case of Mr H, the insurers of a car maker that was still trading, and in the case of Mr J, the Ministry of Defence.

4.10   Mr H: bladder cancer and the car industry

This case involved a gentleman who had worked as a machinist for a large car manufacturer, where he made different components of the suspension of cars such as the Morris Minor and Marina. I owned a Marina in 1986, probably because I only had £150 to spend, and all I could find for that money was a turmeric (well, sort of diarrhoea)-coloured 1975 model. This car came with a 1.3-L engine (designed nearly 40 years previously), about 10 months (Ministry of Transport vehicle Inspection certificate, MOT) and smelt of advanced decomposition. I ran it for 6 months, and in 1 week, it blew its exhaust off at the manifold, the gearstick came off while I was driving and the trunnions seized, making it nearly impossible to steer. I kept it going largely by removing parts from my friends' dead British Leyland cars. Of course, I had no concept of the full horror of British car ownership until my purchase in 1988 of a 1980 Rover SD1 3500V8, of which, more later.

In the Birmingham area in the 1960s & '70s, major components, such as body panels and box sections, engines, transmissions, differentials and other running gear were all manufactured in specialist plants owned by British Leyland. A further complex network of other companies manufactured components for Leyland, such as Dunlop (tyres) Lucas (lights, dynamos, alternators and other electrical components), Smiths (clocks and speedometers) and Triplex (glassware). Other parts, such as dashboards, upholstery and many other fittings, were made by small local concerns. Then, as today, a car factory supports a complex network of suppliers, and the industry will always be sought after, politically and economically, as well as for those who need employment with it. All the components were then shipped to a main plant where the whole car would be assembled. A car plant is a loud and spectacular sight, and I was hugely impressed with Volkswagen's Wolfsburg Plant, which I toured as a teenager in 1974.

Today, the majority of car parts, as well as many engine and drivetrain (gearbox, axles and differentials) and suspension components are made very cheaply in vast amounts from stampings and mouldings using semi-automated processes. A typical suspension control arm in a modern front-wheel drive car is just a steel stamping with a sealed balljoint and bushing attached. When the balljoint shows signs of free 'play', the whole arm assembly is cheap enough to replace. In the 1960s, suspension and drivetrain designs were such that many essential components were still effectively made by hand, using a variety of milling, cutting, grinding and broaching machines, which were in turn manufactured by large concerns such as Cincinnati, which had a factory in Birmingham.

Drivetrain components have always been made from very hard steels, which have to withstand high stresses, so to cut such metal creates a great deal of heat, which must be dissipated if the cutting tools are to have an economic lifespan. The finished metal can also corrode very quickly, so to arrest that process, to protect the cutting tools, to improve the quality of the finish and to ensure that tolerances were observed, various cutting fluids were used. You may have seen videos of these tools cutting metal in a shower of fluid, which either looks like oil or a milky or coloured substance, known as 'suds'. The cutting heads and/or the metal to be machined would be spinning and setting up such a process, and operating it often caused anyone in the immediate proximity to become heavily contaminated with the splash of cutting oils. Mr H worked in such an environment, carrying out the various cutting, broaching and grinding procedures in making drivetrain and suspension components. In the early part of his career, he was paid by the number of units he manufactured (piecework) rather than an hourly rate. Mr H provided an extremely detailed account of his working experiences, and they corresponded closely to those described for the pre-1980 car industry in Chapter 1. Of course, Health and Safety was not well appreciated in the 1960s and 1970s, and many of the machines Mr H used did not even have guards on them, making them quite dangerous to use. In addition, they were very expensive to buy, so they were rarely replaced and often extremely old and outdated. The cutting oils themselves were recycled endlessly to save money until they were contaminated with bacteria and often smelled appalling.

In retrospect, it is easy to suggest that the operators should have worn gloves, but Mr H explained that some processes are so detailed and 'fiddly' that bulky gloves would make the work very difficult, particularly if a man was under pressure to make as many driveshafts as he could to ensure a good wage. Over the last few decades, latex and thin nitrile gloves have appeared, which can protect hands without affecting dexterity. However, anyone who has worked on cars in high summer will be familiar with the saturating sweat that collects in latex gloves. You remove the gloves and must dry your hands thoroughly, or it is difficult to don the next pair of gloves. This is uncomfortable, messy and time-consuming, so it is tempting to just use your bare hands as the men often did. There were various tricks of the trade, such as rubbing the hands with Vaseline™ before work to make oil easier to remove. The men's overalls were their own responsibility, and they were required to have them washed and laundered themselves. Mr H supplied colour pictures taken of himself and his work colleague in the late 1970s, which clearly showed that their overalls were heavily contaminated. The factories were old, and washing facilities were not usually very extensive in the various factories and toilet breaks often restricted. Even as late as the 1990s when BMW owned Rover, the Germans were amazed to find workers assembling cars whilst standing in pools of water from the leaking roof of one facility.

Mr H's case was a substantial undertaking, and other expert reports were commissioned and submitted on aspects of the oils and the nature of their toxicity, as well as the working environment. Aside from the exploration of causation, my report, as follows, provides some insight into the world of component machining in the British car industry of 1960s, as well as the relationships between the men on the shop floor and their managers.

An Expert report prepared for Birmingham Crown Court by Dr M.D. Coleman on the instructions of **** Solicitors concerning the case of Mr H (claimant) against the Company (defendants).

Expert Qualifications (as before)

Material instructions

Mr H contends that his bladder cancer was associated with his exposure to a variety of different petro-chemical products which he encountered as part of his job as a machinist. I have been requested to provide an expert report on the following aspects of Mr H's case against the Company.

- The agents contained in the oils which are likely to have been the causes of his cancer.

- Determination of the nature of Mr H's exposure to various oils during his work.

- The biological and physiological mechanisms that were part of the process of the development of his cancer.

- The influence of smoking in Mr H's case.

- Was Mr H's cancer foreseeable, did negligence and breach of duty of care occur on the part of the Company?

1. Carcinogenic agents contained in the oils
   It is clear that Mr H was exposed to a considerable number of petro-chemical products during the course of his work at the Company. These have been listed as follows:

   - Unrefined/mildly refined mineral oils

   - Highly refined mineral oils

   - Mixtures of mineral oils and water, known as emulsions or 'suds'

- Synthetic oils of vegetable origin, some containing diethanolamine and nitrite

- Semi-synthetic oils which are a mixture of mineral and synthetic oils

(i) Considering the mineral oils, in the most general terms, refined petrochemicals can be divided into three major groups: straight chain paraffin saturates (non-carcinogenic), alicyclics (cyclic saturates and non-carcinogenic) and aromatic hydrocarbons (carcinogenic). The aromatic content of a particular oil is partly related to the type of base crude oil used, its refining history and the type and severity of any finishing process [8]. The simplest aromatic hydrocarbon is benzene (six carbon atoms in a closed ring) and its single-ring intermediate relatives, xylene, toluene as well as naphthalene (double benzene ring). Multiples of three benzene rings or more called polycyclic aromatic hydrocarbons (PAHs). For the purposes of this report, the term aromatic hydrocarbon can be taken to include all benzene-type derivatives.

(ii) Other agents classed as aromatic amines are also found in very small quantities in non-refined oils and basically benzene or multiples of benzene with a chemical group called an 'amine', which is nitrogen and two hydrogen molecules written as 'NH_2'. The term aromatic hydrocarbon can include aromatic amines, but I will refer to aromatic amines separately. Benzene itself is known to cause leukaemias and other aromatics such as PAHs are known carcinogens of the lung and scrotum. Aromatic amines such as benzidine, BNA and PBNA are established carcinogens and have been specifically identified as bladder carcinogens due to exposure in the 1930s and 1940s in the rubber industry.

(iii) From the Disclosure, it is not possible to identify accurately all the different oils to which Mr H was exposed during his working life. However, it is certain that he was in regular contact with aromatic hydrocarbons and aromatic amines which were known human carcinogens. Synthetic oils are only thought to be a risk if they contained amine-based additives. Aromatic hydrocarbons are practically insoluble in water, and they may make up to 10–20% of crude oil and up to 40% of some unrefined mineral oils. The cancer risk associated with all these compounds is related to degree of exposure and quantity of agents present in the various oil combinations that were employed in the metal cutting processes.

(iv) In the study of the risk of cancer in animals, an individual chemical's carcinogenicity can be determined with a high degree of accuracy as this is the only chemical involved in the study. This option is not open in human studies where groups of individuals are followed as they are exposed to a variety of different agents over many years. The compounds involved, the amount of exposure and the conditions of the workplace are not under the control of the scientists writing the reports, and of course the authors are totally reliant on the statements of the workers and the factory records to determine which agents or groups of agents were involved. In addition, processes which occur during high temperatures may form hundreds of other unknown compounds of varying risk.

(v) Aromatic amines are, as previously stated, an established cause of bladder cancer. It has been suggested in the past that bladder cancer due to mineral oil exposure has been caused by the presence of aromatic amines in the oils, either naturally occurring in the oil or added later as an antioxidant [9]. Although the use of aromatic amines in industry has been gradually reduced, recent reports indicate that the risks of bladder cancer have not commensurately reduced for workers in various industrial occupations. Indeed, some current literature suggests that exposure to PAH is a significant risk factor in bladder carcinoma. Pesch et al. [10] have evaluated the risks of bladder cancer in response to a number of chemicals, including various aromatic hydrocarbons as well as aromatic amines. This work involved 1000 cancer sufferers and 4200 controls. The PAHs emerged as a strong bladder cancer risk factor, even after adjustment for smoking histories. Indeed, in this study, PAHs were a greater risk than aromatic amines. Among many other reports, bladder cancers in furnace workers in a Steelworks in the United States were linked to PAHs [11]. These data suggest that PAHs themselves may be another cause of bladder cancer, whether or not they contain aromatic amines.

(vi) The other major group of toxins to which Mr H was exposed includes nitrosamines. Synthetic cutting fluids were introduced in the 1950s mainly to impart post-machining corrosion resistance to ground steel surfaces. These contain mostly water, along with nitrite and an amine such as diethanolamine or triethanolamine, plus a variety of other agents such as emulsifiers and biocides. The nitrite and amines were intended to act as antioxidants, prevent corrosion and improve the finish of the machined component. Unfortunately, in the high temperatures present at the cutting surfaces, the antioxidants react together, and the resulting compound, N-nitrosodiethanolamine (NDELA), is carcinogenic to animals and probably to man [12, 13]. This possibility was first discovered in the 1970s, and up to 3% of cutting fluids could contain agents such as NDELA [12]. It has been estimated that a machine operator using cutting fluids which contain NDELA-like compounds may excrete 40 µg (0 millionths of a gramme) daily, in urine, indicating considerable exposure [14]. Smoking is also a major source of carcinogenic nitrosamines, although a recent estimate of exposure to tobacco-related nitrosamines put exposure at between 1.5 and 6 µg daily [15], substantially less than that might be encountered through cutting fluid exposure.

(vii) Overall, nitrosamines are certainly animal carcinogens as mentioned earlier, and humans react similarly to these agents in terms of how the toxins behave in the body [16]. Interestingly, chewing tobacco yields more than fivefold higher nitrosamine levels compared with cigarettes, and this form of tobacco usage is associated with a very high incidence of mouth tumour formation [17]. As a definitive study cannot be carried out where direct dosage of humans occurs with these compounds, it is not possible to prove beyond doubt that nitrosamines are human carcinogens, but since they are so potent in animals and they react with human DNA [18] in a similar fashion to that of animals, it would be foolhardy not to assume that they are human carcinogens.

(viii) It may be concluded that the balance of probabilities suggests the routine handling and exposure to oils with even minimal aromatic hydrocarbon, aromatic amine or nitrosamine content would increase significantly risks of cancer compared with the usage of oils free of the agents mentioned earlier.

2. Nature of Mr H's exposure to carcinogenic agents

(i) There are a number of reasons why many agents are carcinogenic. Firstly, they must be capable of specifically damaging DNA in a way that does not destroy the cell. The damage must be subtle enough for the repair mechanisms of DNA (rather like a constant motorway maintenance team) to miss or not be able to keep up with. Normally, major DNA damage would be spotted, and the cell would be dismantled in a manner that minimises the leakage of toxic entities into the rest of the body, rather like the removal of asbestos from an old building. If damage is so subtle that the repair systems miss it, then the damage becomes part of the person's DNA, that is, 'self'. This means that the change in a gene or its control systems will be propagated through future cellular generations. If this gene is faulty and departs from bodily control, a cancer may eventually result.

(ii) If a chemical is capable of causing this scenario, it must firstly reach the cells. If it is very soluble in water, it could not pass through undamaged skin. If it was breathed as a vapour or mist, it might be absorbed into the lungs, but it may not enter cells very efficiently once in the blood because the cells have membranes which are barriers to water-soluble agents. The most dangerous carcinogens are the most soluble in oils and fats, as not only can they pass through skin and blood, but they can also enter the lungs from aerosol mists very efficiently and, once in the blood, pass easily into cells. Once inside the cells, they can be biochemically changed to toxic carcinogenic substances.

(iii) Mr H was exposed to mineral oils, mixtures of oils and water (suds) and synthetic oils, all of which contained various oil-soluble carcinogenic agents such as aromatic hydrocarbons and aromatic amines, as well as some water-soluble agents such as nitrosamines. Most of these chemicals can penetrate the body relatively easily through the lungs and skin. Areas such as the scrotum are particularly vulnerable to such chemicals, as the scrotum is 80-fold more permeable to oils than skin on the hands or feet. The nitrosamines could enter via the lungs and possibly the scrotum; certainly as far as lung penetration is concerned, if the droplets of the mists containing the nitrosamines are 5 μm in diameter or less, this would promote absorption.

(iv) Certainly, if the skin was damaged by cuts, for example, penetration of all these toxic agents would be accelerated, and those in manual labour are particularly prone to such damage. The route of entry of the carcinogens is only relevant in terms of the efficiency of one route over another. More oil is likely to enter the body through breathing an airborne mist compared with skin contact. Oils entering the lungs would be partly trapped by the cilia, tiny hairs which protect the lungs by wafting toxins trapped in mucous up the bronchial tree to be coughed up into the stomach and thence the digestive system.

(v) The oils would enter the circulation in the same way as dietary fats. In the case of the 'suds', or mixtures of mineral oils and water, the risk from aromatic hydrocarbons and aromatic amine carcinogens in the oil fraction of the mixture would still be present, although it would be correspondingly reduced compared with that of pure mineral oil.

(vi) The oils with which Mr H was working would have been continuously present in his body throughout his working life at the factory. A number of the working processes he describes indicate that he was heavily exposed to various oils on many occasions and would have been breathing oil mists which contained droplets as well as oil-related combustion products in the atmosphere of his workspace.

(vii) It is also worth noting that amongst the most volatile fraction of an oil, that is, the most easily evaporated and capable of travelling through the air are the aromatics (benzene and amine derivatives), which are the carcinogenic fractions of the oils. Mineral oil-induced cancer study was well established in the scientific literature from the 1920s onwards and was present in the Company management mindset from the early 1960s, along with knowledge of how easily these toxins would enter the body. However, Mr H was not protected from exposure to these agents to any consistent and meaningful degree.

3. Physiological mechanisms of the cancer development

(i) Generally, the repair mechanisms described in the previous section can protect DNA from damage for many years. Indeed, it is possible to withstand a considerable length of exposure to damaging or 'mutagenic' chemicals without any cancer developing. However, if the exposure is for a particularly long duration and the chemical, such as a nitrosamine or an aromatic hydrocarbon damages DNA, then our defence mechanisms can let some genetic damage escape correction.

(ii) Mostly, DNA is such an enormous molecule that such damage may have little or no consequences. Unfortunately, there are some genes that can cause serious problems if they are damaged. This can lead to cells ignoring internal commands to live or die, and uncontrollable cell division can result. The resulting tissue mass is now effectively beyond the body's control and may become a tumour. Cancer may also result from changes caused in 'oncogenes'. These genes are usually only operative during uterine development to orchestrate the explosively rapid growth required necessary in a foetus. The control mechanisms, such as the oncogene 'off switch', can be damaged by a mutagen, causing tumours to appear, sometimes many decades after the original exposure to the mutagen.

(iii) The reason why a cancer arises specifically in the bladder and not some other part of the body is due to the chemical nature of the agents to which Mr H was exposed as well as the site of exposure. Aromatic amines and hydrocarbons are not by themselves damaging to DNA. However, they are recognised by the liver, which chemically alters them to make them more soluble in water so they can be eliminated in urine. This process of chemical change which occurs in all our livers is called metabolism, and it means that the agents are subject to a high-energy chemical enzyme 'sledgehammer' which does make them more water soluble, but makes them less stable also. In the same way, a child knows no different than to hit a piece of metal or a live grenade with the same force, the process of liver metabolism can unwittingly create unstable and mutagenic chemicals.

(iv) The liver can deal with this problem with a second process which links a very water-soluble molecule, called a glucuronide, onto the toxic agent. The result is called a conjugate and is now very water soluble, safe and will be excreted in urine. The liver itself is well defended against cancer, and hepatocarcinomas are rare in Western countries. Inside the conjugate, the toxic chemical remains, but it is temporarily shackled to the water-soluble chemical. The conjugate then leaves the liver, and through the bloodstream, it reaches the bladder.

(v) The environment of the bladder is not conducive to the stability of the conjugates, and enzymes cause the conjugate to break down, releasing the toxin to attack the bladder, which is delicate and poorly defended compared with the liver. In working environments, men often do not drink enough fluid, and their urine becomes concentrated, and infrequency of urination means that the toxins are in contact with the bladder mucosa for long periods of time. Indeed, even low fluid intake by itself predisposes the bladder to cancer. Thus, the reactive and dangerous metabolites have plenty of opportunity in a concentrated state to cause the damaging cancerous events, which were described earlier.

4. Influence of smoking in Mr H's case

(i) Mr H has admitted having an intermittent smoking history. It is undeniable that there is an association between bladder cancer and smoking. The most recent studies indicate that the risk of developing bladder cancer is threefold higher in smokers compared with non-smokers. Interestingly, a smoker is nine times more likely to die of lung rather than bladder cancer. This is probably due to the relative rarity of bladder cancer (the 11th most common cancer), and even as a smoker with no occupational history of exposure to other carcinogens, it would be statistically less likely to develop bladder cancer, compared with other cancers.

(ii) Many of the toxic agents in cigarette smoke are also present in cutting fluids such as aromatic hydrocarbons and amines, as well as NDELA-related nitrosamines. However, there are a number of factors that suggest that tobacco usage was a smaller contributory factor to the development of his condition, compared with his occupation. Firstly, as mentioned in section 1 of this report,

Mr H's exposure to tobacco-sourced nitrosamines was likely to be considerably lower than to synthetic cutting fluid–sourced carcinogenic amines. This is mainly because breathing air laden with nitrosamines and aromatic amines throughout the working day is likely to lead to much greater quantities of the toxins to be consumed compared with moderate cigarette use.

(iii) In addition, Mr H's total exposure to tobacco-sourced carcinogens was substantially reduced during the 9 years of his working life when he had ceased to smoke. It can be suggested that the relationship between smoking and occupational bladder cancer may be no more than additive. It is useful to note that in studies such as those previously cited [10], the carcinogenic potential of occupational exposure to aromatic hydrocarbons still emerges despite the smoking histories of the patients analysed. On balance, my opinion is that smoking in this case was a material contributory factor, but the major factor was exposure to aromatic hydrocarbons, amines and nitrosamines.

5. Foreseeability of Mr H's cancer

Mineral oils

1. It is reasonable to suggest that the foreseeability of whether workers would develop cancer hinges on the knowledge of their degree of exposure to known carcinogens during their work. Mineral oils in general had been known since the 1930s to cause increased risks of cancer in several industries. Aromatic hydrocarbons had been known to be carcinogenic since the 1930s from experiences with the cotton industry, and Vol. 4 of the Disclosure, Document 103, (28.11.69) indicates that the Company was well aware of this work. Three years prior to Document 103, Document 17 shows that several reports were written in 1966 to address the health concerns regarding mineral oils in machine shops in the Company.

2. Document 17 echoes these reports and recommends that only safe non-carcinogenic white oils should be used although there was doubt over the availability. This document shows that the white oils were tested and found to be acceptable but 'not cheap'. The increased cost would be £500 per month. Two years later, this progressive informed position had changed and had been watered down. Document 103 restated that the Company knew that the aromatic hydrocarbons were the problem and that ideally, they should be absent and only white oils used.

3. This was deemed impractical due to the high volumes of oils required in the car industry. The net cost increase was not mentioned, but the factor of £500 per month mentioned earlier must have been taken into consideration in the final decision. The document then underlines the 'next best quality oil' would be solvent-refined product, which had a much reduced aromatic hydrocarbon fraction.

4. This document underlines that the aromatic fraction should be no higher than 12%. It must have been clear that the oils used in the 1950s and 1960s contained far higher aromatic contents. Document 21 of Vol 4 (14.11.69) shows that one of the Company's cutting oil suppliers was very concerned at the levels of aromatic

hydrocarbons in their previous products and had been working for some time to reduce them.

5. Between April and June 1969, Burmah-Castrol introduced increased solvent refining to reduce aromatic levels in Magna BD and CF oils. Documents 101–105, Nov. 1969–Jan. 1970, underline the high aromatic levels found in Forward machine oils (Document 105 showed one of these oils to have 23.1% aromatics), which were then used, and Project 7028 was set up to replace the Forward oils with Ilocut oils (482- and 106), which were less aromatic and therefore safer. There are numerous examples of oils submitted for use in the plant failing to meet with approval due to their aromatic levels exceeding 12% (such as in Document 101). In addition, Document ref CL 5795 refers to the testing of the aromatic hydrocarbon content of Sulfcut 105 from Duckhams (21.5.70), and it indicates an intention to monitor aromatic hydrocarbon content in oil to preserve the 12% maximum.

6. This shows that from 1969, the Company was well aware of the long-term risks of exposure to aromatic hydrocarbons in cutting oils; they knew that they had to actively minimise these risks, and there is evidence that they were attempting to institute procedures to ensure that high–aromatic content oils were not used. However, they had considered using aromatic-free oils but had rejected this in favour of the arbitrary 12% limit. This decision appears to have been made on the grounds of cost, despite the suitability of the oils and their health benefits. Document 84 (Vol. 4) shows that the Company knew that the adoption of solvent-refined (lower aromatic) oils would not remove the cancer risk; it 'only reduces it'.

7. From Volume 2 of the Disclosure, a Factory Safety sheet dated 11.2.70 discussed the proposed use of Ilocut 482 and mentioned that repeated skin contact could develop into cancer. It emphasised that skin contact should be minimised. My reading of this situation is that from 1969 to 1970, even if lower–aromatic content oils were used, a substantial and acknowledged risk remained to the workers handling these oils.

8. There are no apparent scientific or medical criteria which support the adoption of the 12% aromatic content limit. It is not clear from the Disclosure why this value was decided upon and who took the decision. Possibly, it was believed that a reduction from, say 30% to 12% would reduce the risk commensurately. Unfortunately, it is apparent from the Disclosure that even the 12% limit was sometimes disregarded. Tudor oil contained 12–14% aromatics, Quaclad 252 contained 19.1%, Clearedge contained 20–24% and Sulfcut 105 was over 12% also. As late as 1983, Magna BD oil contained 21.8% aromatics. In 1979, a data sheet from Duckhams shows oils available that exceeded 14% and 23% aromatic levels (Core Documents, Literature Search). These levels are after refinement, although it is difficult from the Disclosure to ascertain how widely through the Company's different plants these oils were used.

9. In the early 1970s, the cancer risks from Ilocut 201 were known by the Company, as was its propensity for causing dermatitis. Also in 1970, it was realised belatedly that catalytic 'cracking' occurs at tool tips, increasing oil aromaticity and that

recycling of various oils (they were expected to be used for 12 months in some cases) increased aromaticity also. This was in spite of the recommendations of the Society of Occupational Medicine that recycling was not a good practice.

10. It is therefore clear that Mr H will have been exposed to a large number of various aromatic hydrocarbons from 1957 to 1982. In addition, the aromatic oil contents would have been increased by some Company practices even though by 1970, the Petrochemical Industry and the Company were aware that the cancer risks of oils were in direct proportion to the aromatic contents of the oils. In my opinion, the risk of Mr H and his colleagues developing cancers was foreseeable and preventable.

'Soluble' oils (emulsions/suds)

1. In the early 1970s, it was clear in the scientific literature that nitrosamines were potent animal and likely human carcinogens. By 1976, the US Government recognised that nitrosamines could be formed from additives in cutting fluids. Suppliers of fluids such as Sunbeam Anti-Corrosives were willing from 1977 to replace nitrite-containing fluids with nitrite-free fluids (Core Bundle, document 330, Dr K – letter to Mr Q). A memorandum from Mr Q states that the Company were using nitrites and amines in its cutting fluids in 1977, and some form of response to the US information should be initiated as the situation could become 'almost as emotive as asbestos' (Core Bundle, document 331).

2. The meeting on 10 May 1977 (Core Bundle, document 332) was 'made aware of the current information available from the United States, Europe and the United Kingdom and the action taken by the relevant authorities'. The consensus was that 'none of the evidence confirms that a pathological health risk had been proven at this time', although the Company did restrict any further additions of nitrite-containing cutting fluids to the inventory.

3. The Company Safety Advisor stated that the allegations were based on 'very slim data' (document 335). The Advisor seemed more concerned that the shop floor personnel should not gain 'advantages' from inferring health risks (document 335). Prior to 1976, I feel the Company cannot be held accountable for nitrosamine risk incurred by the men working in their factories, as there was no official evidence of a problem. Once a US Government organisation published its concerns (which were not under any circumstances based on 'very slim data') and then their own suppliers took this warning seriously, the Company should have taken the risks seriously.

4. Therefore, by choosing not to act as other organisations and their own suppliers were acting at the time, the Company did not appear to consider the safety of its workers as a high priority. This attitude had not changed by 1979, when much more scientific data were available. It is likely that Mr H would have been exposed to carcinogenic nitrosamines during this period; even if he did not specifically use them himself, the substances will have been breathable in the air surrounding the machines.

5. Degree of negligence and/or breach of duty of care at the Company

(i) The Disclosure indicates that the Company knew of the relationship between cancer and mineral oils, which had been researched in the 1920s and 1930s. From 1962 to 1970, it was aware of the various genital cancers that were linked with mineral oils. Clearly, protection from the oil in terms of physical splash onto the skin and inhalation of mist would be of paramount importance considering the Company's knowledge of the risks involved. Complaints about oil fumes were made in 1964, and it was known by the Company that ventilation was inadequate at least 2 years before that date.

(ii) Mr Z (a former work colleague of the claimant) in his statement felt that there was never any real ventilation until he retired in 1987. In the Defendant's lay witness evidence, there is some confusion as to whether there was any active or merely passive ventilation of the shop floors. Certainly, most of the Defendant's witnesses (X,Y,Z and W) refer to oil mist/haze as being constantly in evidence, especially in the Bar-Auto areas. However, most witnesses denied that it was a problem, and it was 'nothing to worry about'. The Company Doctor in his statement stated that he felt that oil haze was only a problem if it was visible, and medically it was not of any significance. This is a rather surprising point of view for a Company Doctor, especially such a senior figure. If this was a supposedly medically informed view of the possible hazards of oil haze, it suggests that there would be little management impetus to solve what was actually not even recognised as a problem. X and Y in their statements concede that the only time the oil haze was not present was when the workers were on holiday.

(iii) As stated earlier, oil haze is a combination of respirable droplets and combustion products; it would have been clear in the 1950s that high levels of atmospheric haze would be hazardous to health over a considerable period of time of exposure. The Company Occupational Health Advisor, in one of his contributions to a Conference on Health Hazards of Cutting Oils mentions that cutting and grinding machines were often bought by the Company to cut at one speed but were actually operated at twice that speed and coolant flow to extract more productivity from it. Indeed, he conceded that this process promoted the coolant mist problem, and 'we are sometimes our own worst enemy'. If a large number of machines were operated (up to 100 units in the Bar-Auto Shop) beyond their designated and intended capacity, it would be apparent that the oil haze problem would be exacerbated.

(iv) From 1960 through to 1966, the Company were reluctant to adopt impermeable overalls as it did not believe that they were a viable alternative to regular cotton overalls, which were clearly inadequate as protection. By 1966, the Company Safety Officer was aware that the men were wearing their overalls too long and that they were 'excessively' contaminated. The level of contamination is clearly disputed by many of the Defendant's witness statements, which state that heavy contamination was rare and workers thus contaminated would be asked to wash and were sent home.

(v) The statements of Mr H's work colleague and the widow of another colleague support the extent of high oil contamination that it was possible to experience, after cleaning the machines at the end of the week. It is interesting that one of the nurses, Mrs H, in her statement had seen enough cases of cutaneous reactions to oil and suds contamination to clearly delineate between the types of rashes formed by these coolants. She did mention the high level of oil contamination of some workers.

(vi) The Company was also aware of the high cancer rates in certain plant areas such as the auto shop, and a visiting Company Doctor had noted the high levels of oil mists and the cancers. In 1966, workers were worried about press articles over cancer in car factories, and they were reassured by the Company. In 1967, The Institute of Petroleum recommended that oil-impermeable overalls be issued to the workforce, and adequate washing facilities be made available. There is again conflict regarding the Defendant's lay witness statements, where most mention that impermeable overalls were available and were also worn on a regular basis. From 1966 to 1975, the Company tested and rejected many designs of impermeable aprons on many grounds, some of which were clearly cost based.

(vii) The men were denied 'Multithene' suits as they were too expensive. The Company had known for most of Mr H's working life at the plant that conditions were not protecting the men from contamination from substances that were known at the time to be carcinogens. The Company did appear to try to alleviate conditions after 1970, but in 1974, foremen were complaining that regular examinations of the men were not being carried out. This seemed to be a combination of the voluntary nature of the examinations and the lack of cooperation of some of the men. Even if the men were uncooperative, the examinations should have been carried out.

(viii) The excessive amount of time that was taken in the development of practical oil-resistant aprons was inexcusable, given that the Company had known for decades that scrotal cancer was a risk from oil contamination due to lack of clean or impermeable overalls. The Company should have insisted that the men wear them. As late as 1970, showers and towels were not available to the men as this was 'not practicable'. Again, this was disputed by the Defendant's lay witness statements. By the late 1970s, there were still complaints about the contamination of filtration machines, and it was likely that the oils were not being properly cleaned as a result. Strangely, the men were also asked not to wear gloves with certain machines on the grounds that the gloves would become internally contaminated and the oil would be close to the skin. This may have been the case with absorbent gloves, but impermeable nitrile gloves had been available commercially for years.

(ix) Mr H's statements comment on the large quantities of oil which contaminated his arms, hands and overalls. Colour pictures from the core documents support the case that the men's overalls were clearly heavily contaminated, around the midriff/genital area. As late as 1987, on one particular occasion, the level of oil contamination at the XXXX factory (Vol. 4, Disclosure, Report GOH 912, 22.7.87) was recorded to be severe. The staircases/wells to the hydromation plant were so oily that it was actually hazardous to enter for fear of slipping on the oil. It was thought on that occasion to be impossible to enter the area without being contaminated with oil. Although it was not possible to say that this was the normal level of oil contamination, the report stated that 'as visible and unpleasant tasting aerosol of coolant mist is present'. For this area, respiratory protection was recommended by this report. It is apparent that there was abundant opportunity for cutting oils to constantly contaminate men via the skin and inhalation routes.

6. Opinion

The Company had long been aware that oils that were used in the 1950s–1960s were carcinogenic, and it investigated the possibility of removing this risk by using white oils which were carcinogen free, but this was not followed through. This was in spite of the evidence that the white oils would have been suitable for the tasks that the mineral oils fulfilled. It is possible that this specific decision, for which no documentary evidence was made available, was taken on the grounds of cost. To minimise the known risk of mineral oils, the 12% level for an aromatic maximum content was introduced, but not always followed. The Company also knew that the aromatic content of the oils would increase during normal work, and the process of recycling and operation of the machines at higher-than-intended capacities all accentuated the risks of these oils to the workforce. The Company displayed no urgency regarding protective measures for the men, and several measures increased the risk to the men.

7. Final summary

The Company failed to protect its workforce through the following failures:

(i) Non-replacement of known carcinogenic mineral oils in the mid to late 1960s

(ii) Failure to adhere to internal procedures regarding aromatic and amine content of various oils

(iii) Very slow replacement of carcinogenic NDELA-containing oils in the mid to late 1970s

(iv) Lack of protection from oil mist/vapours and splash leading to excessive contamination

(v) Failure to prevent increased oil carcinogenicity through excessive recycling

M.D. Coleman,
Lecturer in Toxicology

4.10.1 Case comment

This case was legal aided and cost tens of thousands of pounds and was in process for several years. As you can read from the report, considerable numbers of witness statements were collated on both sides, as well as the other experts' reports; indeed, the experts were initially by no means unanimous in their views on causation. Of course, the central problem regarding causation was trying to mount a convincing argument that something other than an 'accepted' single chemical, such as BNA, was responsible for Mr H's cancer. His exposure to amine-based cutting fluids could well have contributed to his disease also, but it was very difficult, if not impossible to ascribe causation to one or two chemicals. In the 1960s, about half of adult males smoked, and in many cases, the claimant's tobacco consumption is an issue that needs to be confronted, although it must be stressed that it is not a barrier to claiming. I did feel it was necessary to try to compare the possible exposure of toxic agents from smoking, to that of the occupational exposure. Such arguments were not tested in court, and assessing the risk of cancer from a series of chemicals derived from different sources is rather speculative at best, but it does provide a platform upon which to try to estimate exposure/risk relationships.

The report does establish that Mr H was in contact with a large number of potentially carcinogenic agents and that these agents could plausibly have caused his condition and that the Company should have made more effort to reduce the risk, given what they undoubtedly knew about the dangers of the oils. In other areas of the factory where Mr H did not work, unrefined oils were used in various processes such as cleaning machinery and some casting processes, which contained up to 30% aromatics, so the mineral oil aromatic problem was widespread. I do feel that the case for Mr H's personal repeated contact with the oil would have stood up in court, so the combination of high contact with agents that the Company knew in the mid-1960s were carcinogenic could well have been successful. The Company was also slow to pick up on the problems emerging with the amine-based cutting fluids, so its assimilation of contemporaneous safety concerns was sub-optimal, to put it mildly.

Regarding the Company's knowledge of the carcinogenicity of the mineral oils, in the Disclosure, there was a long paper trail of documents which obligingly charted the process whereby the possibility of substituting these toxic poorly refined mineral oils with white oils was discussed. The one document that was missing was the one that officially rejected the white oils on the grounds of cost. This particular 'smoking gun' was perhaps too much to hope for, but it was clear from the document trail either side of the missing article that the Company could not face the cost of these oils and neither could it support the purchase of protective measures like gloves and overalls. The figure of £500 per month mentioned as the increased costs of white oils over mineral oils in the mid-1960s probably adjusts to around £7500 for 2013. However, for a major manufacturer selling in excess of 170,000 cars annually, this seems at first glance a relatively small sum.

To place this somewhat bizarre parsimony in historical context, by the early 1970s, a series of mergers led to Rover, Jaguar, Triumph, Morris and Austin effectively existing under the same management and sometimes even competing with each other for different markets. The resulting sprawling British Leyland Empire included more than 200,000 workers and 48 factories. The industry is now extinct in terms of British ownership, and it is not remembered fondly. However, it should be remembered that in terms of vehicle design, the British car industry pioneered the small, transverse engine, front-wheel drive platform which is ubiquitous today, but revolutionary for its time, when the vast majority of cars were rear-drive with north–south engine configurations. Again, the designers of my wonderful Rover SD1 in the early 1970s, for example, were tasked with producing a new car which was the same weight as its predecessor, the Rover P6, but with features such as the latest laminated windscreen and stainless steel bumpers. The elegant new car was duly delivered within 35 lb of its target weight, although its build quality was staggeringly bad. After a considerable amount of remedial mechanical work, my SD1 V8 was quick, smooth and thanks to a compact and effective manual transmission designed for the Triumph TR7, quite economical. However, it remained grotesquely unreliable, and whilst it could accumulate and retain some fluids in quantity (rainwater), other rather more important fluids leaked away from multiple sites (oil, antifreeze, brake fluid, power steering oil) extremely rapidly, no matter how much I worked on the car.

From a business perspective, things were no better. The one really brilliant and innovative design the British car industry produced, the Mini, was underpriced to the extent that whilst over five million were made from 1959 to 2000, the car made no real profit. Ford executives bought a Mini in the early 1960s, dismantled it and then carefully estimated its production costs; they realised that it cost more to make than its sale price. It is of course more than possible to make money in the car industry; Ford (USA) was making five-figure profits on each of their somewhat agricultural Explorers as late as the 1990s. For the British car industry, chaotic management which was way out of its depth, combined with lack of investment in new models and ferociously dire industrial relations, led to the production and marketing of a series of truly appalling cars that were nothing less than calculated mechanical insults to their customers. Regarding the Austin Allegro, more than 640,000 were built, although the customers responded by scrapping 99.96% of them as of May 2013 [19]. It is unknown as to how many of the 291 survivors listed on the UK Driver and Vehicle Licensing Agency (DVLA) database might actually move under their own power.

Prior to the start of the court case, it was clear that Mr H's health was not likely to be robust enough to sustain the effort involved. The two sides reached an agreement, and Mr H was paid £168,000 in compensation. This was the culmination of 8 years of effort, yet around half the money disappeared very quickly, taken by debts incurred by Mr H's failed business venture started after he had left the Company and of course the benefits agency demanded a certain amount of money to be returned. However, Mr H had fought a long, valiant and heroic battle in spite of his health, and his victory in the case was highly significant for those who had been injured by their work in the car industry.

The legacy of such a case is effectively the automation of pretty much all the dangerous processes in car building as well as the transformation of the working environment in the form of purpose-built plants which are advanced, efficient and, above all, safe to work in for many years. Ironically, under foreign management, this transformed industry now sees British workers manufacture cars equal to and sometimes exceeding even Japanese or German build-quality standards.

4.11   Mr J: Bladder cancer; crankcase oils and diesel

If you are one of those people that find cars and weapons overpoweringly interesting, then tanks will be frankly irresistible. From a scientific perspective, the really interesting aspect of this case for the author was the role of diesel emissions and their links to bladder cancer. As mentioned previously, the expert report writer should be impartial and balanced; however, I have always had a particular visceral loathing of diesel and diesel engines of every type, and I find it fascinating that modern diesel engines can apparently pass apparently stringent Euro emission regulations, yet they still emit black smoke when they start, as well as during hard acceleration, which would disgrace a pre-World War II steam engine. The high sulphur content in UK diesel causes particularly nauseating and acidic emissions, which make streets unpleasant places to be during heavy traffic. I recall a rather fatuous debate in the United States arose a few years ago over 'what kind of car would Jesus drive'. Given his only documented and rather brief use of transport involved a borrowed and somewhat modest steed, it seems unlikely that Jesus would own a car at all. However, it was obvious to me that when none of Satan's fleet of battered white vans was available, the Evil One would be racking up very high mileages in either an Austin Montego Countryman Diesel Estate, or possibly a heavily overloaded, rock-spewing, smoke-belching tipper truck on a very tight schedule. Diesel engines are perceived to be good for the environment, but their nitrogen oxide, PAH and particulate emissions are decidedly bad for humanity [20].

The following report concerned the effects of diesel emissions combined with exposure to crankcase oil suffered by a gentleman who had spent his working life driving and maintaining tanks in the British Army. It is instructive to climb into a tank and imagine what it is like to spend a whole day or night in one, and there are so many opportunities to crack one's head against something very solid even when the tank is stationary. In a combat situation, such as in World War II, the jolting, the deafening roar of the engine and a mounting and fully justified sense of vulnerability if you were in any other tank but a German Tiger makes you have a healthy respect for all tank crews. Tanks of all designs have always been known for their mechanical fragility as the desire to protect the crew with as much armour as possible meant enormous weight, which wore out engines and transmissions extremely rapidly. Consequently, they need constant servicing and maintenance to keep them mobile. German tanks of World War II were the most technically advanced in the conflict, with a single Tiger 1 requiring almost as many man hours to produce as an entire U-Boat. Indeed, German attention to detail seen in their cars today is nothing new; unlike their Russian and American counterparts, German tank workers paradoxically even took the time and trouble to hand grind smooth rough armour edges.

Unfortunately, even the large petrol engines they used, such as the 690 hp V-12 Maybach in the Tiger 1, were not powerful or reliable enough to provide the required battlefield agility. The Russian T-34s used more rugged and economical V-12 diesels, although these were hampered by dreadful air filter designs; indeed, build-quality issues in the rest of the T-34 were legion, and they leaked so badly that heavy rain would short their electrical systems.

After the war, diesel engine propulsion for tanks gained favour in European designs, probably not least because of the problems the Germans had running out of petrol at crucial moments in campaigns. Unfortunately, given the state of diesel engine technology after World War II, moving a 55-tonne object at serious speed across the countryside would create some fearsome and highly visible diesel emissions, and so it proved until relatively recently.

Mr J started his military career as a tank mechanic, working more or less constantly to maintain large battle tanks, often literally in the field in Germany, as part of the British Army on the Rhine (BAOR). He developed bladder cancer in his mid-30s, which is extremely young for such a condition to emerge. It was apparent that he had been exposed to several possible sources of carcinogenic oils, but again, there was little if any evidence of specific bladder carcinogens such as aromatic amines. He did become exposed to some very carcinogen-rich diesel emissions in the course of his work with the tanks, but he also had much greater contact with used crankcase oils, which, most amateur mechanics and scientists will tell you, are full of pungent tarry residues that are extremely rich in PAHs. Together, these exposures I felt would be strong candidates for causation of his condition, so I was confident that an effective report could be assembled.

RE: An Expert Report prepared by Dr M.D. Coleman concerning the possible occupational causality of the malignancies suffered by

Mr J (d.o.b. XXXX)

Expert qualifications (as before)

Material instructions

Mr J, the claimant, has described how he was exposed to excessive amounts of oils, lubricants and toxic automotive emissions during his service with the British Army (1971–1990). The claimant alleges that this high level of contamination with toxic petrochemicals encountered during his service was the major causative factor in the development of his bladder cancer in 1989 and its subsequent reappearance in 2008. The bladder malignancy had spread to the left kidney, which necessitated extensive surgery involving the removal of several organs and tissues including his bladder and left kidney. The supplied Histopathology report (Dr M--, 15.04.08) stated that the spread of the malignancy appears to have been halted. It is likely that such major surgery would have a permanent and substantial impact on Mr J's quality of life.

I have been asked by XXXX Solicitors to report on the factual basis for a causal link between Mr J's exposures to toxic petrochemicals during his military service and his bladder cancer.

Context and nature of Mr J's exposure to petrochemicals

From the statement supplied to me made by Mr J, as well as a pictorial record of some periods of his service, it is clear that his occupation as a tank driver and mechanic has led him to a particularly intense and consistent physical contamination with the various lubricants, coolants and emissions from the Chieftain tanks he was, according to his account, effectively 'living in' during his periods on active service or on exercise.

Wider context of his occupation

1. The Chieftain tank was part of a post-war tank development programme borne out of the very high losses sustained by Allied Armour in engagements with technically superior German Tigers and Panthers towards the end of World War II. Ironically, the Chieftain, in service from 1966 to 1995, shared the German design emphasis on gunnery and protection, but also unfortunately also shared their mechanical fragility. The sheer weight of tanks in general (the 1960s' Chieftain was actually 2 tonnes lighter than a World War II Tiger) has always caused rapid component wear, which in turn necessitates the need for constant mechanical attention from individuals such as Mr J.

2. It is clear that Mr J's account of the legendary unreliability of the 19-L, two-cycle, 750-horse vertically opposed six-cylinder L60 Leyland engine is corroborated strongly in military literature; indeed, some overseas recipients of large orders of Chieftains later demanded that the L60 engines should be replaced with a more reliable and less maintenance–dependent power plant [21]. The design of the L60 engine was dictated by the perceived military necessity of minimising restrictions on the type of fuel which could be used, to prevent or alleviate shortages. The Chieftain L60 was designed to run on virtually any fuel, including fuel oil, diesel, kerosene, petrol or a mixture of these [21]. Consequently, its design promoted high fuel consumption and emissions, as well as a lack of reliability. The multi-fuel concept is still used in some US Military vehicles to this day, unfortunately accompanied by similar reliability problems.

Comparison of contamination level with the author's experience

1. Mr J's account of the high level of contamination he experienced is actually much more severe than in other cases I have dealt with, such as in the automotive industry. In car factories, contamination in machining, grinding, boring and milling processes involved exposure to oils used for cooling and lubrication. Although these oils up to the mid-1970s contained a number of potential carcinogens, they were freshly obtained from refineries and had not been exposed to any combustion processes, which dramatically increases the carcinogenicity of the oil. Mr J was contaminated by engine oils which had been exposed to combustion in an engine, which even by the standards of its time was extremely polluting and inefficient.

The visible emissions from Chieftains were so high that they were considered a military liability as they revealed the tank's positions to the enemy. Mr J's account of the start-up procedure of several tanks in large hangars also demonstrates a very high exposure to the most polluting period of a diesel engine's operation, where partial combustion led to the production of very high levels of visible aerosols (smoke).

2. In the car industry up to the mid-1970s, physical exposure to oils was direct, as well as through contaminated overalls which had to be washed by the men or their families. However, it is noteworthy that there was an opportunity for the men to remove their overalls at the end of the day when they returned to their homes. While Mr J was on exercise in his tank, he was unable to adequately wash or decontaminate himself. Therefore, his net exposure to contaminated engine oils and coolants was significantly higher than in men who developed bladder cancer in the automotive industries.

3. Although it is anecdotal, in my experience, the cases I have dealt with in the automotive industry have been in men who have worked for a period of around 15–35 years, and the average age they developed their cancers was in the mid-50s. In most cases, they were smokers, which is the primary contributing factor in the development of bladder cancer. Mr J developed his cancer at the extremely unusually early age of 36. This may have been linked with the high level of contamination he encountered as well as the length of time the oils were in contact with his skin. In the automotive industry, test operations of engines were sometimes carried out, producing fumes within confined spaces. However, this level of atmosphere contamination appears to have been much less than encountered by Mr J's experience of several 19-L engines operating at low efficiency in a relatively confined space.

Routes of absorption into the body

1. Aerosols from diesel engines contain a vast range of aromatic hydrocarbons, as well as particulates. Aromatic hydrocarbons are very soluble in oils (lipophilic), and consequently they can enter human cells easily. The volatile aromatics are directly absorbable through the lungs, whilst the heavier multi-ring polycyclic aromatics (known as polycyclic aromatic hydrocarbons or PAHs) are usually associated with the particulates, but can still enter lung cells. Both types of aromatic agents can be relatively easily systemically absorbed (enter the body) so that they have access to all the organs of the body through the blood supply. Diesel engines of the 1960s and 1970s were particularly inefficient and produced visible emissions which contained very high levels of PAHs, which are unacceptable and illegal today.

2. Engine oils and lubricants are also highly lipophilic, and when they have been exposed to combustion, they also contain various volatile aromatic hydrocarbons which can be inhaled or absorbed through skin as well as the lungs. Transdermal absorption is most efficient in the scrotum, due to the high surface area of the skin in that area and its high permeability, which is up to 80-fold greater than other skin areas [22]. Clearly, the lack of the ability of Mr J to remove or change

contaminated overalls during military exercises would contribute to the absorption of various aromatic hydrocarbons in the oils via the scrotal sac. Indeed, the longer the skin is left contaminated, the greater the systemic absorption.

Other factors which affect the toxicity of the oils

1. In the automotive industry, anecdotally, in previous cases, it has been clear that men working in hot oily environments were also restricted in their access to fluids. This was compounded by the propensity of most working men to consume caffeinated drinks such as coffee or tea. These drinks promote dehydration due to their diuretic effect. The combination of restricted access to fluids and the exposure to diuretics tends to cause a concentrating effect in urine, which leaves the products of the body's metabolism in contact with the bladder mucosa for longer periods in high concentrations.

2. These products are highly significant in their ability to cause malignancies (see later section). Mr J would have been subject to the same restrictions in his role as a member of a tank crew, as tanks of the 1960s and 1970s were not air-conditioned as they are today. Pre-1990s' tanks were poorly ventilated, and opportunities for breaks are restricted in military exercises. Poor fluid intake as an exacerbating factor in the development of bladder cancers has been recognised in several occupational studies [23].

Bladder cancer aetiology

1. Bladder cancer is listed as the ninth most common human cancer, with around 250–360,000 new cases diagnosed annually [24]. The 5-year survival from initial diagnosis is currently listed at around 50%, so Mr J is more fortunate than many patients with this disease. It is accepted that the primary cause of bladder cancer is cigarette smoking, which still accounts for more than half of the cases [25]. Estimates vary as to the proportion of the second largest cause of the disease, occupational exposure. This has been listed as between 10% and 20% of diagnoses, and the strong male bias in the sufferers (3.5 men to every woman diagnosed) is accepted as an indicator that this cancer has a particularly strong association with occupation [26].

Causes of occupational bladder cancer: Aromatic amines

1. Historically, bladder cancer was first ascribed to occupation as far back as 1895 in the dye industry through the use of colour-fast aniline dyes [26], and the cancer risks in the rubber industry were detected before World War II. By the mid-1950s, the causative chemical class of agent had been confirmed to be aromatic amines, particularly benzidine and BNA, as well as several other aromatic amine derivatives, such as a component of the dye direct black, 4-aminobiphenyl [27]. Aromatic amines were used in industrial contexts to prevent oxidation in materials, often at considerable levels (up to 1% in rubber) to soften it and prevent it from becoming brittle over time. Various other related amines, aromatic and the

much less toxic aliphatic derivatives, were used in the petrochemical industry to prevent oxidation and deterioration of fuels, lubricants and coolants from the 1950s onwards [28, 29].

2. By the end of the 1940s, production of BNA had ceased in the United Kingdom, and by the end of the 1970s, production had ceased worldwide. As these aromatic amines are formed during the tobacco pyrolysis, they are accepted as the causative agents in bladder cancer linked with smoking [26].

Other causes of occupational bladder cancer

In spite of the removal of aromatic amines from the workplace, in terms of additions to fuels and lubricants over the past 40 years, several occupations are still listed as at higher than normal risk of developing bladder cancer. These include workers in the aluminium industry, where smelting with heavy grades of fuel oil (coal-tar pitch volatiles) is routine. The next highest risks are possibly those in the paint industry, followed by workers in transport, such as bus, train and taxi drivers, as well as selected groups of workers such as salt miners [30]. Two options are apparent in causation: firstly, somehow known causative agents such as aromatic amines are still present in occupational contexts through some mechanism, and they are present in concentrations capable of causing malignancy in the bladder, despite their virtual banning from the workplace. Secondly, scientifically speaking, it cannot be assumed that there is only one group of chemical causative agents of bladder cancer, so there may be other agents in the workplace which are causative.

Persistence of aromatic amines in occupational contexts

1. It is established that aromatic amines are formed through the burning of organic material such as that in tobacco use [25]. However, it is also clear that the burning of fuels also forms heterocyclic aromatic amines which are chemically the same as proven bladder cancer carcinogens such as BNA [27], which are also found in diesel fuel emissions; these agents are mutagens in that they can damage DNA and they are capable of causing cancer in the same way as BNA [31–34].

2. Mr J was heavily exposed to engine and lubrication oils, which were extremely contaminated with pyrolytic products such as heterocyclic amines, which are highly mutagenic [33]. Indeed, diesel emissions from fossil fuels are much more mutagenic in the Ames test compared with synthetic (vegetable oil) fuels [35]. Mr J was also exposed to high levels of diesel emissions, which contain mutagenic aromatic amine derivatives.

Role of PAHs in bladder cancer development

1. Over the last 30 years, it has been suspected that other closely related chemicals to aromatic amines are capable of causing occupational bladder cancer. The exact causative agents in this disease are difficult epidemiologically to locate, as human populations contain many confounding factors, such as individual susceptibility, different working conditions and durations of exposure, as well as tobacco usage

[24]. It is characteristic of the scientific literature that studies often show a clear relationship between smoking and bladder cancer, due to the known presence of BNA in tobacco smoke [25, 36]; however, other causes of bladder cancer have been less well documented.

2. The common link between the current high-risk occupations for bladder cancer (aluminium smelting, painting, transport industries) is PAHs derived from the combustion of fossil fuels, particularly heavy oils and diesel. The links between PAHs emitted from diesel fuel combustion and bladder cancer have been controversial. Experimentally, models of the human bladder have demonstrated the carcinogenicity of PAHs [37], and several studies have indicated that PAHs in diesel emissions are linked with human bladder cancer in occupational contexts [38, 39]. However, other studies failed to demonstrate a causal link [40–42]. However, it has been shown recently that exposure to diesel emissions are associated with increases in the levels of known human bladder carcinogens such as BNA, which was detected in the urine of salt miners [30]. In addition, a recent meta-analysis of many occupational and epidemiological studies carried out by the Health and Safety Executive has indicated that PAH exposure has a causal link with bladder cancer [43]. Since a meta-analysis is a comprehensive evaluation of many studies in an area with regard to an attempt to answer a specific question within stated conditions, this finding is very significant. The authors were careful to place their findings in context. They stated that

> There was also an association of PAH with bladder cancer .... but this finding was less robust than that for lung cancer, being largely dependent on two studies of aluminium production workers [43].

They also stated that

> Bladder cancer is also much less common than lung cancer, especially as a cause of death, so lung cancer is reasonably considered as the lead risk [43].

3. In effect, this suggests that high exposure (such as that encountered in aluminium smelting) to PAHs is a causative link in bladder cancer development, although in terms of risk the 5-year survival for lung cancer is only 5%, whilst for bladder cancer, it is eightfold higher. So the relationship between PAH exposure and lung cancer is stronger than that of PAHs and bladder cancer in terms of the risk of death, rather than necessarily actual causation.

In the context of this Expert Report, the Health and Safety Executive (HSE) report and other reports support the role of PAHs in the causation of Mr J's condition, as his exposure to PAHs, through contaminated engine oil, hydraulic fluid and high levels of diesel emissions, absorbed through multiple routes into his body, suggests that PAHs as well as exposure to mutagenic heterocyclic aromatic amines were the major causative factors in the development of his bladder cancer.

Professor M.D. Coleman

4.11.1   Case comment

Soon after the report was complete, the news came from a specialist barrister that this case came under the Armed Forces' immunity to prosecution for any negligence or specific circumstances which could have been responsible for an ongoing medical condition if those circumstances occurred before 1987.This meant that I had the extremely difficult task in trying to link Mr J's condition with a very narrow window of exposure that he had, which was after 1987 to the end of his service, when the exposure ceased. I did not feel confident that this would be tenable, but I felt I should try to address the questions posed by the barrister in the following addendum.

RE: An Addendum to the Expert Report prepared by Prof. M.D. Coleman (dated June 26) concerning the possible occupational causality of the malignancies suffered by

Mr J (d.o.b. XXXX)

Updated material instructions

Further to a recent communication with Ms X and a teleconference with Mr X, a barrister from XXXX Chambers Bristol, it is now apparent that the Crown Immunity (Armed Forces) Act 1987 applies in this case, and the only admissible timeframe which could be considered as relevant to toxin exposure, which may be linked with Mr J's subsequent condition, is from 15 May 1987–December 1988.
    Two questions arise:

1. Whether his previous (now unactionable) exposure (1973–1980) had already set in motion an irreversible chain of events which would have led inexorably to the development of his cancer.

2. Whether Mr J's exposure to tank exhaust fumes during this period as detailed in his statement could be responsible for the development of his cancer.

Background: Cancer development in tissues

Cellular changes

Cancers are effectively autonomous tissues which no longer accept normal bodily control. More than a century of scientific and medical research has not yet uncovered anything like all the steps in this complex process. Carcinogenesis has for many years been conveniently resolved into two major, if incompletely understood, stages. The first was termed initiation, the second, promotion. Initiation is the process whereby an external or internal agent causes some form of change in the genetic control of a cell, which does not in itself inevitably lead to a cancer.
    This could be a mutation in DNA sequences, or a change in chromosomal disposition without a mutation, which is a new area recently explored known as epigenetics. Initiated cells do differ from other non-initiated cells in that they live longer and can be resistant to toxicity and hormonal and chemical instructions issued by other cell systems. They cannot normally be detected as different from other cell systems.

Promoters are usually chemicals that generally act to cause initiated cell populations to break free from their existing programming and begin to grow without restraint. Promoters are not carcinogenic to normal tissues.

Occupational toxin effects

Occupationally, a carcinogen such as tobacco, used crankcase oils or diesel emissions is likely to contain a wide and complex combination of different initiators and promoters. In the case of Mr J, he was exposed to two of the aforementioned agents in the 1970s, and in the 'window' between 1987 and 1988, he was exposed to diesel emissions.

Response to question 1

As detailed in the Expert Report of 26 June, there are several substances in diesel and used oils which may have acted as initiators and promoters during Mr J's service. However, what is not generally understood is at which point initiation and promotion might occur or not occur in a given period of exposure. This variability and doubt is reflected in the wide range in the individual periods of exposure to carcinogens, which are required to induce a neoplasm. This may range from as little as 5 to 15 years [27, 44, 45] and may also involve a gap of more than 29 years before the neoplasm actually appears [46]. It is also noteworthy that in occupational settings, the vast majority of individuals who are exposed to the carcinogenic agents do not develop the disease. Hence, it is not possible to pin down when initiation and promotion actually take place in the timescale of bladder and other cancers. There are so many events which may take place during initiation and promotion, including patient genetic susceptibility, inhibition and activation of tumour suppressor genes and other risk factors which predispose to bladder cancer, such as being male.

Perhaps a crude analogy to whether or not these events may lead to a cancer might be found in old films of criminals trying to break into combination safes which contain several 'tumblers'. If, for example, eight out of the required nine tumblers have fallen into place, then the safe will still not open, and the criminal will not know how many more need to fall.

The process of chemically mediated DNA mutation occurs constantly and is accelerated in the presence of diesel emissions and used crankcase oils. However, repair mechanisms act constantly also and over any given period of time the persistence and efficacy of an individual's inherited mutation defence systems may or may not be overwhelmed, depending on their inbuilt resilience. With cigarette smoking, for example, the cessation of exposure to the toxins in tobacco will reduce the risk of cancer dramatically, and the risk is measurably lower after only 1 year [47]. Hence once the exposure ends, there is every chance that the individual may dramatically change his cancer 'destiny'. This is also relevant to Mr J's case, as although he did not smoke, it is thought that the same agents which cause bladder cancer in cigarette smoke are present in diesel emissions and used oils.

It is therefore impossible to be certain that Mr J's exposure up to 1987 condemned him inexorably to develop his cancer. Indeed, up to the beginning of 1987, there was no detected clinical sign of the disease, and in the absence of further exposure, it is possible his condition may have been delayed in onset or even not occurred.

Response to question 2

Over 1987 and 1988, diesel emissions appear to be the only agents to which he was exposed. If events prior to 1987 are not relevant to the initiation and promotion of cancer in regard to exposure of diesel emissions, then it is necessary to explore the possibility as to whether both initiation and promotion could conceivably occur in short space of time with regard to diesel emissions.

The major carcinogenic components of diesel emissions are aromatic hydrocarbons, which include aromatic amines. In occupational studies with various groups of workers, such as hairdressers exposed to aromatic amines in dyes, it was shown that a period of exposure was required to be at least 5–10 years [46]. Other studies report exposure periods of up to 15 years [44]. Diesel emissions as a sole cause of bladder cancer is an issue which has not been comprehensively explored. This is partly because exposure to diesel emissions is so variable, ubiquitous and difficult to measure accurately as so many other sources of pollution contain similar toxin components [48]. In terms of recorded durations of exposure to diesel emissions alone which may lead to cancer, there are little detailed data regarding bladder cancer.

However, there is a strong precedent for chemical exposure over short periods leading to bladder cancer, which is essentially the same type of cancer that is developed due to occupational carcinogens. The anti-cancer drug cyclophosphamide is used to treat other conditions aside from cancers, such as the otherwise fatal condition Wegener's granulomatosis. Cyclophosphamide is a well-established cause of bladder cancer [49, 50], and the likelihood of developing a malignancy is dependent on the dose of the agent used to control Wegener's disease and the duration of therapy. In some cases, the initiation of cyclophosphamide therapy and the appearance of a bladder malignancy can be as short as 7 months or as long as 15 years [49–51].

Summary of opinion

• With regard even to current knowledge of cancer neogenesis, it was certainly possible, but not inevitable that Mr J would develop bladder cancer up to 1987, given the degree of exposure he suffered to the various chemical agents with which he came in daily contact.

• The usual range of latency of bladder cancer regarding occupational exposure with respect to aromatic amines and cigarette smoking is from 5 to 15 years of exposure. As the scientific literature is sketchy on diesel emissions and bladder cancer, the author found no specific reports, which described an exposure period of less than 1 year where bladder cancer resulted from occupational exposure.

• However, there is a precedent for chemical agents to initiate and propagate carcinogenesis within the short window described for Mr J's exposure, such as that spanning May 1987 and December 1988.

• Therefore, it is not beyond the realms of possibility that heavy exposure to diesel exhaust could have led to a malignancy in the case of Mr J.

M.D. Coleman,
Professor of Toxicology

4.11.2 Further comment

Essentially, it was very difficult if not impossible to assign causation to the narrow window available, and an opposing expert could argue that the irreversible changes in Mr J's bladder probably had begun before 1987, although again, it is impossible to be certain. Either way, Mr J's case could not progress. He has, however, used his vast knowledge and love of tanks to restore successfully various World War II armoured vehicles, including an example of the legendary Tiger 1, model number 131, which is in full working order.

4.12 Summary

There is evidence in the scientific literature that in many industries, agents other than aromatic amines, such as PAHs or nitrosamines, are mutagenic and could be linked with various cancers, including those of the bladder [52–55], although this remains tough to prove due to the very long latencies seen in this condition. Certainly, it has become extremely difficult to link cases with exposure to the classical aromatic amine bladder carcinogens such as BNA in the engineering and automotive sectors. However, with sufficient exposure, combined with negligence in the provision of protection, it can be argued that bladder cancer malignancies can be attributed to PAHs and other amines.

Interestingly, it might be thought that perhaps the only profession where bladder cancer related to occupational health might still be relatively easily causally related to aromatic amines is probably in hairdressing, due to the azo dyes, which are still used in this area [56]. This is in contrast to the risks for women who dye their hair themselves, which fortunately appear to be much lower to the point of statistical insignificance, with the exception predisposing factors such as acetylation status [2, 57].

References

1. http://www.cancerresearchuk.org (accessed on 11 November 2013).
2. Burger M et al. Epidemiology and risk factors of urothelial bladder. Cancer Eur Urol. 63, 234–241, 2013.
3. Coleman MD. Dapsone: modes of action, toxicity and possible strategies for increasing patient tolerance. Br J Dermatol. 129, 507–513, 1993.
4. Cancer Research UK. http://www.cancerresearchuk.org/prod_consump/groups/cr_common/@cah/@gen/documents/generalcontent/treating-bladder-cancer.pdf, 2013 (accessed on 11 November 2013).
5. American Cancer Society. http://www.cancer.org/acs/groups/cid/documents/webcontent/003085-pdf.pdf, 2013 (accessed on 11 November 2013).

6. National Toxicology Program. Report on carcinogens, 12th edition. U.S. Public Health Service National Toxicology Program, Department of Health and Human Services, Research Triangle Park, 2011.

7. Coleman MD. Human Drug Metabolism: An Introduction, 2nd edition. Chapter 6, Wiley International, Chichester, UK, pp 360, 2010.

8. Health and Safety Executive. The Carcinogenicity of Mineral Oils. Guidance Note. Environmental Hygiene Series, EH58. HMSO, London, 1990.

9. World Health Organisation, International Agency for Research on Cancer (IARC) monograph. Mineral oils (lubricant base oils and derived products). In: Polynuclear Aromatic Compounds, Part 2. Carbon Blacks, Mineral Oils and Some Nitroarenes. IARC Monographs on the Evaluation of Carcinogenic Risk of Chemicals to Humans, vol. 33. International Agency for Research on Cancer, Lyon, 87–168, 1984.

10. Pesch B et al. Occupational risk factors for urothelial carcinoma: agent specific results from a case control study in Germany. MURC Study Group, Multicentre Urothelial and Renal Cancer. Int J Epidemiol. 29, 238–247, 2000.

11. Mallin K et al. A nested case–control study of bladder cancer incidence in a steel manufacturing plant. Am J Ind Med. 34, 393–398, 1998.

12. Loeppky RN et al., Probing the Mechanism of the Carcinogenic Activation of N-Nitrosodiethanolamine with Deuterium Isotope Effects: In Vivo Induction of DNA Single-Strand Breaks and Related in Vitro. Chem Res Toxicol. 11, 1556–1566, 1998.

13. Health and Safety Executive. Nitrosamines in synthetic metal cutting and grinding fluids, Guidance Note EH 49, HSE Books, 1987.

14. Spiegelhalder B et al. N-nitrosodiethanolamine excretion in metal grinders. IARC Sci Publ. 84, 550–552, 1987.

15. Spiegelhalder B et al. Environmental exposure to tobacco-related NNOC. Presented to the 13th annual ECP symposium, London, 1995.

16. Preussman R. Carcinogenicity and structure activity relationships of N-nitroso compounds. A review. Drug Dev Eval. 16, 3–18, 1990.

17. Hecht SS, Hoffman D. The relevance of tobacco-specific nitrosamines to human cancer. Cancer Surv. 8, 272–294, 1989.

18. Dittberner U, et al. Cytogenetic effects of N-nitrosodiethanolamine (NDELA) and NDELA-monoacetate in human lymphocytes. J Cancer Res Clin Oncol. 114, 575–578, 1988.

19. Wilkinson L. UK's top 20 'endangered family cars' revealed. www.telegraph.co.uk/motoring/news/10056212/UKs-top-20-endangered-family-cars-revealed.html (accessed on 13 May 2013).

20. Lean G. Why is killer diesel still poisoning our air? *The Daily Telegraph*, 19 July 2013. http://www.telegraph.co.uk/motoring/green-motoring/10190942/Why-is-killer-diesel-still-poisoning-our-air.html (accessed on 11 November 2013).

21. Dunstan S, Sarson P. Chieftain Main Battle Tank 1965–2003. Osprey, Oxford, 2003.

22. Wester RC, Maibach HI. Principles and practice of percutaneous absorption, 943–956. In: Paye M et al., editors. Handbook of Cosmetic Science and Technology, 2nd edition. Informa Health Care, New York, 1003 p, 2006.

23. Droller, Michael J, editors. Bladder Cancer: Current Diagnosis and Treatment. Current Clinical Urology. Humana Press, Totowa, 472 p, 2001.

24. Parkin DM et al. Global cancer statistics, 2002. CA Cancer J Clin. 55, 74–108, 2005.
25. Zeegers MP. The impact of characteristics of cigarette smoking on urinary tract cancer risk: a meta-analysis of epidemiologic studies. Cancer. 89, 630–639, 2000.
26. Lilienfeld AM, Lilienfeld DE. Foundations of Epidemiology. Oxford University Press, New York/Oxford, 1980.
27. Baan R et al. Special report: policy carcinogenicity of some aromatic amines, organic dyes, and related exposures. Lancet. 9, 322–323, 2008.
28. Brown JE. Mechanism of aromatic amine antiknock action. Ind Eng Chem. 47, 2141–2147, 1955.
29. Papay AG et al. Lubricating oil compositions of improved rust inhibition. U.S. Patent 3,928,219, 1975.
30. Seidela A et al. Biomonitoring of PAHs in workers occupationally exposed to diesel exhausts. Int J Hyg Environ Health. 204, 333–338, 2002.
31. Kataoka H et al. Determination of mutagenic heterocyclic amines in combustion smoke samples. Bull Environ Contam Toxicol. 60, 60–67, 1998.
32. Manabe S et al. Detection of a carcinogen, 2-amino-1-methyl-6-phenylimidazo[4,5-b]pyridine in airborne particles and diesel-exhaust particles. Environ Pollut. 80, 281–286, 1993.
33. Manabe S et al. Occurrence of carcinogenic amino-carbolines in some environmental samples. Environ Pollut. 75, 301–305, 1992.
34. White PA, Rasmussen JB. Mini review: the genotoxic hazards of domestic wastes in surface waters. Mutat Res. 410, 223–236, 1998.
35. Bünger J et al. Cytotoxic and mutagenic effects, particle size and concentration analysis of diesel engine emissions using biodiesel and petrol diesel as fuel. Arch Toxicol. 74, 490–498, 2000.
36. Kellen E et al. Does occupational exposure to PAHs, diesel and aromatic amines interact with smoking and metabolic genetic polymorphisms to increase the risk on bladder cancer? The Belgian case control study on bladder cancer risk. Cancer Lett. 245, 51–60, 2007.
37. Wolfa A et al. The effect of benzo(a)pyrene on porcine urinary bladder epithelial cells analyzed for the expression of selected genes and cellular toxicological endpoints. Toxicology. 207, 255–269, 2005.
38. Kogevinas M et al. Occupation and bladder cancer among men in Western Europe. Cancer Causes Control. 14, 907–914, 2003.
39. Clavel J et al. Occupational exposure to polycyclic aromatic hydrocarbons and the risk of bladder cancer: a French case–control study. Int J Epidemiol. 23, 1145–1153, 1994.
40. Guo J et al. Risk of esophageal, ovarian, testicular, kidney and bladder cancers and leukemia among Finnish workers exposed to diesel or gasoline engine exhaust. Int J Cancer. 111, 286–292, 2004.
41. Cordier S. Occupational risks of bladder cancer in France: a multicentre case–control study. Int J Epidemiol. 22, 403–411, 1993.
42. Siemiatycki J et al. Occupational risk factors for bladder cancer: results from a case–control study in Montreal, Quebec, Canada. Am J Epidemiol. 140, 1061–1080, 1994.
43. Armstrong B et al. Cancer risk following exposure to polycyclic aromatic hydrocarbons (PAHs): a meta-analysis. Research report 068, 2003.

44. Viera V et al. Spatial analysis of bladder, kidney, and pancreatic cancer on upper Cape Cod: an application of generalized additive models to case–control data. Environ Health. 8(3), 1–13, 2009.
45. Harling M et al. Bladder cancer among hairdressers: a meta-analysis. Occup Environ Med. 67, 351e358, 2010.
46. Miyakaw A et al. Re-evaluation of the latent period of bladder cancer in dyestuff-plant workers in Japan. Int J Urol. 8, 423–430, 2001.
47. Patel AR, Campbell SC. Current trends in the management of bladder cancer. J Wound Ostomy Continence Nurs. 36, 413–421, 2009.
48. Frumkin H, Thun MJ. Diesel exhaust. CA Cancer J Clin. 51, 193–198, 2001.
49. Knight W et al. Urinary bladder cancer in Wegener's granulomatosis: risks and relation to cyclophosphamide. Ann Rheum Dis. 63, 1307–1311, 2004.
50. Pedersen-Bjergaard J et al. Carcinoma of the urinary bladder after treatment with cyclophosphamide for non-Hodgkin's lymphoma. N Engl J Med. 318, 1028–1032, 1988.
51. Talar-Williams C et al. Cyclophosphamide-induced cystitis and bladder cancer in patients with Wegener granulomatosis. Ann Intern Med. 124, 477–484, 1996.
52. Wingren G, Axelson O. Cancer incidence and mortality in a Swedish rubber tire manufacturing plant. Am J Ind Med. 50, 901–909, 2007.
53. Talaska G et al. 2-Naphthol levels and genotoxicity in rubber workers. Toxicol Lett. 213, 45–48, 2012.
54. Chien YC et al. Assessment of occupational health hazards in scrap-tire shredding facilities. Sci Total Environ. 309, 35–46, 2003.
55. Brown T et al. Occupational cancer in Britain: urinary tract cancers: bladder and kidney. Br J Cancer. 107, S76–S84, 2012.
56. Takkouche B et al. Risk of cancer among hairdressers and related workers: a meta-analysis. Int J Epidemiol. 38, 1512–1531, 2009.
57. Koutros S et al. Hair dye use and risk of bladder cancer in the New England bladder cancer study. Int J Cancer. 129, 2894–2904, 2011.

5
Chronic and acute toxicity of herbicides and pesticides

5.1 Introduction

Every year, we use millions of tonnes of various herbicides and pesticides to exert control over thousands of species of plant and insect life that have been deemed undesirable, perhaps because they interfere with our food supply, or they threaten our health or that of our pets. Most of these chemicals have been designed as a result of research into comparative biochemistry, physiology or anatomy; this is essentially the determination of where the 'enemy' plant or insect differs from humans, in which enzyme systems it uses to survive. Once we establish which of these systems to attack, which are both vital to life and unique to the 'enemy', then various chemical and non-chemical agents can be tailored to inhibit these systems whilst hopefully minimising human consequences.

However, it is clear that the idea of a 'selective' toxin or poison is at best naive and at worst completely untenable, partly because such selectivity is very dependent on dosage and our existing and often limited knowledge of comparative biology and environmental degradation. Although we are at the apex of the pyramid of life on our planet, we are nevertheless subject to the same 'rules' as all other life. We use the same fuels, such as food stuffs and oxygen; we use very similar cellular respiration processes and we are all pretty much made of the same components, such as proteins and amino acids, which are made in very similar ways. The sheer complexity of the interdependence of life on earth unfortunately ensures that no toxin is ever really selective, especially at higher doses. Indeed, whilst the observation from decades of genome research that humans share about half their genes with bananas has become an amusing scientific cliché, it is true that we share a common ancestor with fruit flies and almost 80% of human disease genes are found in these insects [1, 2]. In addition, the fruit-fly genome is sufficiently similar to that of man that meaningful extrapolations have been made towards human systems ranging from the genetic control of circadian rhythms, learning and memory, as well as neurodegenerative disease; there are even similarities in fly and human responses to ethanol intoxication [3].

Expert Report Writing in Toxicology: Forensic, Scientific and Legal Aspects,
First Edition. Michael D. Coleman.
© 2014 John Wiley & Sons, Ltd. Published 2014 by John Wiley & Sons, Ltd.

This commonality of all species has led us to the point where many supposedly selectively toxic insecticides at best impair, or at worst eliminate, valuable non-target species such as bees, fish and other aquatic populations [4, 5]. Perhaps the supreme irony in this area is that an herbicide, paraquat, turned out to be one of the most lethal human poisons ever developed and there remains no effective antidote to a lingering and unpleasant death after ingestion of this chemical. Even a passing glance at a container of a 'selective' anti-pest agent of some kind will carry a long list of species that it also kills and various statements to the effect that nobody should breathe the fumes or allow this 'selective' product anywhere near themselves or their pets.

5.2 Herbicide/pesticide toxicity evaluation

Nevertheless these toxic products have to be handled and applied in the environment by a host of different individuals, ranging from trained spray operators and agricultural workers to ordinary people attempting to eradicate weeds from their lawn or fleas from their pet. Consequently, short of searching for a used sealed protective suit with a separate filtered air-supply, some exposure to these toxic agents is unavoidable. The question arises then is how these agents have been judged safe to use. To some extent, this is answered in the regulatory processes which govern the introduction of new herbicides and pesticides. The manufacturer must submit extensive data on how the compound is selective to its target species and approximately how toxic it is likely to be to animals. This latter estimation can be made through simple acute toxicity tests on rats or mice, where the agent is dosed to the point where half the animals die as a result of exposure. This LD_{50} test, as well as data from other tests involving the oral and inhalation routes of exposure, plus measurement of dermal irritation, is all collated and the relative toxicity of the agent classified by regulatory authorities. In the United States, the Environmental Protection Agency (EPA) categorises pesticides using I–IV, where I is listed as a poison, with the usual pirate symbols on the label. The EPA demands that a 'signal word' should be on the label of the agent which describes the toxin. So a category I agent with a rat LD_{50} at or below 50 mg/kg is labelled as 'danger'. Category II encompasses toxicity up to 500 mg/kg and this is listed under 'warning', whilst category III (500–5000 mg/kg) is labelled as 'caution' and IV (5000 mg/kg and above) does not merit even 'caution'.

5.3 Herbicides: Toxicity

Popular perceptions of herbicide toxicity probably originate from two well-publicised toxic agents, the first of which has already been mentioned, paraquat. This, along with its close relative diquat, is a bipyridylium derivative which is a category I human toxin. Given the lack of antidotes and the plethora of safer alternatives, there is no rational explanation as to why these agents continue to be manufactured around the world in quantity. As little as 5–10 mL of concentrated paraquat is lethal to humans and its environmental persistence exceeds 20 years in soil [6]. Paraquat and diquat usage is usually restricted to professional personnel, and in the United States paraquat is supplied as a blue liquid with a strong odour and an emetic added to it as a last ditch protective measure, although it is also highly toxic to skin. It was first marketed in the 1960s by the somewhat gnomically named Plant Protection Ltd, from Bracknell, Berkshire, and it deranges photosynthesis by diverting electron flows and forming cytotoxic free radical species [7]. As to its selectivity, its ability to form large amounts of such species in any living cell means that if something is alive, then paraquat can kill it. In man, it causes destruction primarily of the lungs, oesophagus and the kidneys. Mortality is around 33% and death may occur due to multiple organ and respiratory failure, depending on the dosage [8]. Diquat is marginally less lethal than paraquat although it is not selective for the lungs. Diquat mainly targets the kidneys and the brain; indeed, its neurological effects can be severe enough to cause fatal seizures [9]. Both compounds are used in preparations either together or with other agents, such as diuron. Chronic exposure to bipyridylium agents is also linked with many health impacts, not least of them, severe depression [10].

A second example of an infamous herbicide is 'Agent Orange'. More than 70,000 tonnes of this toxin was used by the US Military in an ecocidal measure to defoliate a substantial area of Vietnam in the late 1960s and early 1970s to reveal National Liberation Front for South Vietnam (Viet Cong) and North Vietnamese Army movements. This was a mixture of two relatively specific anti-broadleaf phenoxy acid herbicides, 2,4,5-T and 2,4-D. Whilst 2,4-D is still being used, 2,4,5-T was banned in 1985. This is because it contained dioxin (2,3,7,8-tetrachlo rodibenzodioxin), an impurity which is a potent toxin and carcinogen. This was formed from two 2,4,5-T molecules reacting together during the second stage of the herbicide's synthesis only if the temperature of the reaction was allowed to exceed 160°C. The subsequent catastrophic and continuing impact on the health of US Military Personnel and, of course, the Vietnamese was only belatedly recognised [11, 12].

Whilst these two herbicides have a grim reputation, surprisingly, the process of exploiting comparative anatomy and physiology has been (with some exceptions) more successful for manufacturers with respect to the differences between plants and animals; indeed, aside from aberrations such as paraquat and 2,4,5-T, herbicides are generally much less toxic than other biocides to mammals, as they target plant-specific processes such as photosynthesis that do not occur in animals. Many herbicides are actually much safer than a number of household agents in terms of their mammalian LD_{50}s [13]. In general, the most toxic herbicides are not easy to obtain for domestic use in the developed world and aside from occasional suicide bids [14] the majority of the agents available are relatively safe if handled with appropriate precautions.

5.4   Case history 1: Mr K and Roundup©

This case involved a gentleman in his thirties who worked for an oil company in a plant where natural gas was treated with ethyl mercaptan to enable its detection by smell. Mr K worked in a control room and was present at the plant when the main gas tanks were sprayed by trained personnel from a commercial pest and weed control concern. Very soon after the spraying he and a colleague reported some chest problems which abated quickly in the case of the colleague, but not with Mr K. His health deteriorated and he developed pneumonia. Approximately one month after the spraying he died in hospital. There was no immediate explanation for his death and no specific organism could be identified which could have been responsible for his illness. As he was relatively young, this was also an extremely unusual occurrence. Therefore, his widow was determined to find out what was responsible for his death. I was asked to explore the possible causation linked with the use of the pesticides Roundup and diuron which were employed during the spraying, as well as other drugs and chemicals that he was exposed to during his last days. The report was eventually submitted to the local Coroner prior to the inquest.

An expert report on the possible causation of the death of Mr K

Expert qualifications (as before)

Timeline of Mr K's illness

The approximate timeline of the events leading to Mr K's death is summarised here.

May 27th: possible occupational exposure to various chemicals. Period of exposure
    and amount of agent involved unknown.
May 28/29th: Mr K was examined in routine medical and concern expressed over his
    chest sounds. He reported symptoms of a chest infection to his wife.
June 2nd–6th: GP prescribed antibiotics.
June 7th–13th: at hospital for treatment with antibiotics
June 13th–25th: at home, but unwell
June 25th: readmitted to hospital
July 1st: worsening condition necessitated admission to high dependency ward
July 2nd: moved to intensive care
July 3rd: death recorded at 11.15 p.m.

From the time of exposure to possible chemical toxins to the time of his death, approximately 36 days elapsed. His death is unexplained insofar as being due to a specific infection or agent.

General summary of the events of Mr K's death

1. Mr K suffered from what was described as an atypical (unusual) pneumonia,
   which caused considerable progressive inflammation and disruption to his lung

function, as well as other symptoms such as an external rash. He was intensively treated with several different antibiotics over the course of the disease and none appeared to arrest the advancement of the condition. His pneumonia caused so much damage to his lungs that they would have released many cellular factors known as cytokines, which can appear when tissues and organs are in extreme metabolic distress.

2. Many of these agents are highly destructive to the function of other major organs such as the kidneys, which in Mr K's case then failed. Once a chain of progressive organ failure is established, it is not unusual for other previously healthy organs to collapse relatively rapidly, leading to death. At autopsy (Dr X's Post-Mortem Report), the lung damage was named as the direct cause of death; indeed, it was so comprehensive that there was 'no area of normal lung tissue'.

Possible causes of the pneumonia

Although a considerable number of potent and usually effective antibiotics failed to save Mr K, it was not conclusively established which organism may have been responsible. However, many of the features of presentation of Mr K's disease were consistent with an infectious agent. In addition, a normal inflammatory reaction will occur in any tissue or organ in response to the presence of bacterial or viral particles and this process itself will be responsible for tissue damage. In some cases, the immune response is more destructive than the initial infection. This is notable in conditions such as hepatitis.

Direct chemically mediated pneumonitis: many agents, both chemical and particulate, can cause direct injury to the lungs, which usually resolves after the agent has been metabolised or otherwise cleared from the tissue. Volatile organic solvents, pesticides, herbicides and reactive particulates such as dusts or asbestos may cause such injury.

Chemical-mediated inflammatory/autoimmune condition: an acute and aggressive immune response can also result from exposure to chemical agents and particulate matter. Usually, once the chemical agent is withdrawn the reaction will cease progressing and eventually subside. In some rare cases, an autoimmune condition is triggered, which possesses its own momentum which is independent of the initial stimulus.

Combination of the aforementioned elements: it is conceivable that initial chemical exposure led to direct lung injury, which was followed by an opportunistic infection and severe immune reaction. Multiple processes may have all participated in the process of initiation and propagation of the atypical pneumonia, which was responsible for Mr K's death.

Instructions

I have been asked to comment on the possibility of the existence of a toxicological component to the causality of the atypical pneumonia that led to the tragic death of Mr K on 3rd July.

Mr K's chemical exposure

Context

1. During the course of Mr K's normal duties at the Liquid Petroleum Gas Processing station where he worked, there was opportunity for exposure to several potentially toxic agents. These include two broad categories of chemical.

2. The first category includes agents which were handled by the machinery at the processing station. These include natural gas (such as butane, propane and pentane) as well as agents involved in the processing of the natural gas which include deodorants and a stenching agent (ethyl mercaptan). Although these agents are capable of causing respiratory toxicity, it appears highly unlikely that Mr K was exposed to them, as an HSE report has indicated that there was a sophisticated detection system for these chemicals present at the facility. In addition, although ethyl mercaptan is well known for its acute toxicity, not only were the detectors in place, but they had proved reliable since 2005 (according to the HSE report). In any case, ethyl mercaptan has such a potent and repulsive odour that the human nose is very sensitive to this agent, so it does not appear like that this chemical could have accumulated in the vicinity of Mr K's workstation sufficiently to cause toxicity without him immediately noticing and reporting the leak. Hence, given the information available, it does not appear likely that LPG or ethyl mercaptan would have been implicated in even chronic mild irritation of Mr K's respiratory system, as leaks would have been detected and repaired quickly.

3. The second group of agents which are most likely to have reached Mr K in detectable quantities include the herbicides used routinely around the site, to reduce the fire risk of dry vegetation around the LPG tanks. This second group of agents includes 'Roundup© biactive' and 'Freeway'. In the supplied literature from the case, it is apparent that Mr K was not working in the vicinity of 'Freeway' (diuron) spraying, so it is unlikely that he was exposed to that agent. Roundup was the main agent used in the area where Mr K was working and this agent has been considered in detail.

'Roundup© biactive'

1. Roundup is marketed in a variety of different versions and they all contain the broad spectrum herbicide glyphosate, usually as an isopropylamine salt, alongside what is termed 'adjuvant' chemicals. The function of these chemicals is to improve the penetration of the agent into plants. There are several adjuvants used in different formulations of Roundup and often the adjuvant used and its concentration is classed as a trade secret and is not always obtainable. However, the commonest agent employed is polyethoxylated tallow amine (POEA).

Roundup acute (immediate) human toxicity

1. Although Roundup and its preparations are often marketed as relatively safe for humans, there is a great deal of evidence that they are acutely and chronically toxic

to man. Acutely, a Roundup preparation is fatal if consumed at volumes of approximately 200–300 mL [14]. Interestingly, Roundup preparations are increasingly involved in suicide attempts around the world.

2. The major effects in Roundup overdose are sore throat, nausea, fever, respiratory toxicity (difficulty breathing) and renal (kidney) failure. If a fatal dose has been consumed, death occurs within 72 hours. There is some evidence that humans are more susceptible to Roundup toxicity than animals. Roundup and its adjuvant agents are very injurious to the throat and respiratory tract mucosa during suicidal consumption [15].

3. There is a wide variety of symptoms associated with acute non-suicidal exposure to the herbicide through skin contact or inhalation of vapour whilst spraying. These include eye irritation, blurred vision, joint blisters, skin rashes, rapid heartbeat and palpitations, elevated blood pressure, chest pains, coughing, headache and severe nausea [16]. There have also been reports on its toxic effects on lung function [17].

4. Although many documented cases involved exposure to considerable contamination due to spillages, as well as deliberate consumption, even mild exposure can lead to severe rashes (sometimes lasting months) as well as dizziness, fever, nausea, palpitations and sore throat [18]. A major part of the acute toxicity of Roundup preparations has been attributed to the adjuvants such as POEA.

Roundup and chemical pneumonitis

1. There is a single report in the scientific and medical literature of chemical pneumonitis attributed to Roundup exposure, which was published in 1998 [19]. In this report, an individual was exposed to a solvent vapour which contained Roundup in a confined space for a considerable period of time. He was admitted to hospital suffering from mild to moderate respiratory distress. There was X-ray evidence that exposure had occurred to both lungs. His body temperature was 1°C above normal and his other vital signs were stable, although he had an irritative cough, shortness of breath and episodes of coughing blood in sputum.

2. The patient was treated with precautionary intravenous Augmentin (used in Mr K's case), as well as steroids and oxygen. He responded well and was discharged in two days. He continued to suffer chest tightness and hoarseness and there was evidence of burns to his airways. His lung function continued to improve, although his liver enzymes showed a very mild increase which took several weeks to return to normal and may well not have been related to this incident. Medical personnel from the manufacturers of Roundup (Monsanto) vigorously contested the role of Roundup in this incident, on the grounds that the droplets generally formed by the agent were too large to penetrate the lungs to any considerable depth [20].

3. The original reporting physicians stood by their diagnosis, which they based on extensive inquiries into the individual's working environment and toxin exposure. It is more than probable that Monsanto will adopt a similar position if they are challenged in this case over the toxicity of Roundup.

Roundup formulation chronic (repeated) toxicity

1. It is well established that Roundup is as toxic if not more toxic to aquatic life compared with vegetation [21] and during chronic exposure, Roundup is more toxic in the presence of the adjuvants than alone [21] and increasing numbers of studies have implicated Roundup in chronic human toxicity. Human cellular investigations have revealed that glyphosate and its adjuvants are endocrine disruptors, damage DNA and are probably carcinogenic, mutagenic and reprotoxic at concentrations which are recommended to be used as herbicides [22, 23]. The nature and mechanisms of glyphosate's toxicity are not fully investigated or understood.

Mr K and Roundup exposure

Level of exposure

1. Mr K's respiratory problems coincided with the use of Roundup in the vicinity of his workstation and it is not unreasonable to suspect his symptoms may have been consistent with exposure to the herbicide and its adjuvants, possibly due to 'drift' of spray. Some of these respiratory symptoms appeared to affect at least one of his work colleagues also, suggesting that two individuals affected at the same time may be more than just coincidence. However, several points must be noted.

   - The HSE report mentions that spraying around the LPG tanks was routine and must have occurred with similar herbicides on previous occasions, yet there do not appear to be any reports of contamination or problems in previous sprayings.

   - Assuming both Mr K and his colleague were both exposed to Roundup, it is notable that the respiratory problems of Mr K's colleague resolved spontaneously, albeit over several days.

   - It is difficult to ascertain if there is any basis to the idea that Mr K should have suffered any heavier contamination of the herbicide than his colleague, despite his tendency to breathe habitually through his mouth.

   - Roundup is certainly chronically and acutely toxic and does show lung and respiratory effects; however, it is again very difficult to ascertain what sort of 'dose' Mr K received. It is impossible to determine whether he was perhaps exceptionally sensitive to the effects of the agent.

   - It is impossible to determine whether Mr K was exposed once to a high degree, or mildly several times. This would depend on the duration and quantity of spraying.

Mr K's disease pathology and Roundup: Role of direct cytotoxicity

1. Assuming Mr K was exposed to Roundup and given that wind conditions were not exceptional over the week of spraying, it is difficult to see that he could have been exposed to anything other than a mild dose of the agent. The patient in Pushnoy's

report [19] was exposed to Roundup in a confined space and was most likely to involve a larger dose of the agent compared with Mr K's exposure indeed, that patient presented with similar symptoms to Mr K (respiratory distress and coughing blood), although his lungs did recover within four days and he was able to breathe without distress or obstruction. However, Mr K's condition progressed and amplified to a fatal result over five weeks.

2. Direct cytotoxicity is seen with some chemically mediated pneumonitis conditions, where sufficient damage is caused to the lungs that irritative cough, sputum production and coughing blood may occur, as was reported in 1998 [19]. Generally, a toxic agent may cause cellular injury from a single dose and once the agent is cleared from the cells (Roundup is metabolised to aminomethylphosphonic acid; AMPA), either the cells survive and recover or they enter necrotic or apoptotic (programmed) death. Provided that the threshold for severe injury has not been exceeded, once the toxin has gone the tissue should recover and any symptoms will subside.

3. There are chemicals such as paraquat and diquat, where the agent is capable of causing continued cell toxicity (through oxidative stress) through a form of toxic recycling known as REDOX-cycling. Paraquat causes a self-sustaining massive tissue damage process which destroys the lungs. There is no evidence to date from the scientific literature that glyphosate or its surfactant/adjuvants can behave like paraquat. Indeed, there is no evidence that paraquat was employed by the contract sprayers at the facility.

4. Hence, from a single mild exposure it would not be expected that an agent such as Roundup could, through direct lung cell toxicity, sustain a gradual, five-week long progressive and destructive process of cellular, tissue and ultimately organ (lung) damage once it had been cleared from the tissue through normal cellular detoxification metabolism.

Mr K's disease and Roundup: Other hypotheses

Infection

1. The pathology of Mr K's respiratory decline showed an inexorable progression which was clearly being 'propelled' by some aggressive process. That the process could not be arrested with a succession of antibiotics does not in any way discount an infectious organism-based disease. There is sufficient clinical experience in fatal antibiotic resistant pneumonias which are not associated with any individual organism that the role of infection cannot be eliminated. Indeed, it is likely that any experienced physician will agree with this statement. Many features of Mr K's condition appear to point towards an infectious agent. His immune response appeared to be strong, with fever, joint pains and green sputum production.

2. He appeared to respond to antibiotic therapy sufficiently to allow the hospital to discharge him after his first admission, although he was clearly still not recovered. The surgeon responsible for Mr K's care of his diverticulitis noted in his report that

on his ward round (11th of June) Mr K's fever was absent. In the statement made by the doctor treating Mr K on re-admission on the 25th of June, examination revealed a mild fever. Six days later when the same doctor examined the patient on his return from leave, it is interesting that he stated that Mr K's fever had settled. This suggests that the progression of the condition had been slowed more than once under the pressure of the different antibiotics to some extent. If the disease was entirely inflammatory in origin, it would not be expected that the antibiotics would noticeably affect it.

3. In addition, there is some evidence that Mr K's immune system was already under some stress prior to his illness, as he suffered from diverticulitis (relatively rare at that age) and on-going viral infections such as shingles, as well as a history of exposure to other viruses (such as Epstein–Barr Virus). This may have contributed to Mr K's abnormal susceptibility to the disease process that killed him.

Chemically mediated immune response

1. As mentioned previously, the immune system's response to infection can be as destructive as any infectious organism and there are cases where chemicals can induce immune responses which can be extremely damaging, leading to pneumonitis and the appearance of extensive pulmonary damage which results in bronchiolitis obliterans organising pneumonia (BOOP). It appears that these cases may arise from exposure to a variety of stimuli, from particulates to organic solvents. However, once the patient has been isolated from the trigger agent and after this agent has either been metabolised or has otherwise been cleared from the lungs and other tissues, the situation resembles the progression of acute direct toxicity. The lungs may either sustain irreversible damage which is lethal or they may recover. The process of lung damage does not normally progress for several weeks after the single exposure of the agent.

2. For a pathological process to generate its own disease momentum which is independent of the original 'trigger', an autoimmune process could theoretically have arisen. There are several disease states where drugs may induce immune attack on a tissue, which in some cases may continue long after the drug has been withdrawn. Examples of these conditions include anticonvulsant syndrome and drug-induced lupus erythematosus. These conditions are disseminated (affect several tissues) and often focus their most damaging effects on a single organ. This is usually the liver, because the concentration of enzymes is greatest, which can form toxic metabolites from a given chemical. These toxic metabolites can cause damage to the organ, which attracts the attention of the immune system, which interprets the damage as it would an infection and directs the full force of its cellular destructive systems on that organ.

3. Hence, such reactions do strongly resemble the effects of an infection, such as fever, chills, joint pains and rashes and they are often treated erroneously as infections, when large doses of steroids or other immunosuppressives are actually required. However, this is not unreasonable, as the use of steroids to suppress the immune system when a severe infection is present can be lethal very quickly, so

until infection is ruled out, immunosuppression is not deployed. In the case of anticonvulsant syndrome, the pattern of response is reasonably well known clinically and steroid therapy is usually initiated as soon as there is no apparent 'response' to the antibiotics.

Roundup and an immune response

1. For Roundup and its adjuvants to cause a progressive condition which resembles a chemically mediated immune-mediated destruction of the lung, the chemical would have had to damage the lung in such a way as to initiate immune attack. This type of reaction is already quite rare (anticonvulsant syndrome occurs in less than 1:4000 individuals). For the condition to become a self-sustaining autoimmune process, that is, independent of the significant presence of Roundup and its chemical adjuvants, is even rarer. Roundup is capable of causing rashes and allergy responses and it can also decrease lung function and cause breathlessness and coughing [24]. However, there is no scientific or medical literature precedent for Roundup causing such a devastating and sustained reaction as occurred with Mr K.

2. There are other factors which make it unlikely that Roundup sustained Mr K's pneumonia.

   - Although Roundup can cause rashes and allergies, most serious autoimmune conditions occur after repeated exposure, as the immune system usually requires considerable sensitisation to mount such a devastating and disseminated response. However, it is not clear how many occasions Mr K was exposed to Roundup.

   - The only other report of pneumonitis as a result of Roundup [19] showed both lungs to be affected; whilst Mr K's right lower lobe was a focus of the inflammatory reaction. It could be suggested that an infection would have been more likely to cause this than a chemically induced immune response, which would be distributed more widely across the lungs.

   - The long timeframe (five weeks) over which the disease was capable of progressing is not typical of the general pattern of chemical pneumonitis.

Opinion summary: Role of Roundup in Mr K's death

- On balance of probabilities, the evidence presented suggests that Mr K probably was exposed to Roundup spray 'drift' to some degree and it is likely that it did cause some respiratory symptoms and mild respiratory damage.
- On the strength of the evidence presented and the scientific literature on Roundup's toxicity, I do not believe that this chemical was responsible for the sustained progressive and ultimately lethal pneumonia suffered by Mr K.
- It appears that there may have been certain aspects of Mr K's immune function which may have rendered him especially susceptible to the pneumonia which was probably an unidentified infectious agent or even agents.

- It is conceivable that the initial respiratory insult caused by Roundup could have provided an opportunity for the fatal infection to establish itself in Mr K's respiratory system. This possibility could be explored by consultation with an appropriate specialist in the area.

Other drugs and their effects on Mr K

Salbutamol

1. Mr K was treated with a wide variety of drugs during his illness. Aside from several antibiotics and analgesics, he was also treated with salbutamol to dilate his bronchial tree and improve his breathing. This β-adrenoreceptor agonist operates by stimulating the receptors which relax the bronchi. These receptors are also present in many other tissues and even from an inhaler considerable quantities of a drug may enter the bloodstream either through the bronchi themselves or via droplets of the spray which condense on the throat and are swallowed.

2. The drug may affect other tissues around the body which possess the same receptors and this can typically cause the heart to speed up (tachycardia), breathing to become abnormally fast (tachypnoea), plus effects on blood acidity. The more drug is taken into the body, the more pronounced these effects will be. Different patients display different drug sensitivities and it is possible that Mr K was more sensitive to salbutamol than others. His symptoms suggest either higher than normal sensitivity to the drug, a greater intake of the drug, or both.

3. Despite salbutamol's effects which appeared to have been distressing for Mr K and his family, I would not have thought that the drug would have had any bearing on the organ damage and multiple failure which was caused through different processes which were not likely to have been affected by salbutamol, which is considered a safe drug which remains in wide use [25, 26].

Benzalkonium chloride

1. There is a considerable scientific literature on the tendency for the preservative in many salbutamol inhalers (benzalkonium chloride; BAC) to cause bronchoconstriction (chest tightening and impaired ability to breathe). It is possible that Mr K may have been sensitive to this effect. Bronchoconstriction from inhaled BAC is cumulative (the more the patient is exposed, the more likely it is for an effect to occur), prolonged, and is directly linked with how sensitive the patient's airways may be normally [27–30].

2. However, again, it is unlikely that this effect, unpleasant as it was, had any underlying influence on the main progression of Mr K's illness. It is significant that none of the medical reports made available to me made any discussion of the problematic effects of the salbutamol on Mr K in relation to the progression of his main condition. If they had felt that it might have had any influence on Mr K's outcome, they would have been bound to address this issue.

Michael D. Coleman, Ph.D.
Professor of Toxicology

5.4.1   Case comment

This case involved an invitation (backed by the threat of a summons) for me to appear at the local Coroner's Court. This type of court [31] is conducted by a local council-appointed judicial officer, the Coroner, who is usually medically or legally qualified. The purpose is to investigate a violent, unexplained, sudden or unnatural death, to establish what transpired and how the death might have occurred. Prior to the hearing, the Coroner will have investigated the death and ordered a post-mortem to shed more light on the specific causes of the death. The hearing will most likely not involve a jury and the Coroner will question witnesses, although representatives of the bereaved can also ask questions. The possible verdicts the Coroner can reach include natural causes, accident (misadventure), suicide, lawful or unlawful killing, industrial disease, narrative, or an open verdict. Mr K left a widow and two young children, so from their point of view, the most favourable verdict to take the case further would probably have been an 'open' or 'industrial disease' verdict. There would then have been no barrier to the mounting of a civil case against either the employers of Mr K or the manufacturers of the herbicides involved. The Coroner painstakingly explored all the available aspects of the case, questioning the medical staff responsible for Mr K's care in detail, as well as the family legal representatives and myself, as to possible causality linked to the herbicides. Hence, issues related to the strategy of Mr K's care were investigated vigorously as well as the causes of his pneumonia and death.

The Coroner decided that on balance, the cause of death was essentially one or more infections, rather than a consequence of the spraying, leading to a verdict of natural causes. Whilst it is often assumed that an infection can be easily identified, hospitals cannot always isolate the organisms responsible in the timeframe available in a serious and acute illness and this makes it difficult to select the appropriate antibiotics to treat the problem. In any treatment of an infection, the patient's immune system is effectively being supported by the antibiotics, and a combination of resistance and problems linked to Mr K's immune function *in extremis* probably overwhelmed him.

5.5   Pesticide action: The nervous system

A clearer and more present danger to humans is the chronic and acute toxicity caused by exposure to insecticides, as insects are of course much closer to us than plants and as mentioned earlier in section 5.1, we share more characteristics with insects than we generally realise. There are a wide range of approaches to incapacitating or killing any target insect. There are toxins that affect energy metabolism (rotenone, arsenicals and dinitrophenols), pheromones which impact behaviour and even bacterial toxins. However, the quickest lethal method is to attack and disable the insect's command and control of itself, that is, its nervous system. Animals and insects possess a central nervous system (CNS, or brain) which controls behaviour and a peripheral nervous system (PNS) which gathers sensory information for the CNS whilst executing its commands to facilitate survival and propagation. The most basic unit of both systems is the neurone itself. This specialised cell expends a great deal of energy, pumping sodium ions out and drawing potassium ions in, making it effectively at rest like a long and highly negatively charged battery. When the nerve is stimulated, the sodium channels open all along the neurone length like little gates and the sodium ions rush in, whilst potassium rushes out through its gates and a reverse of potential impulse progresses extremely rapidly along the nerve cell, which is then 'depolarised'. Once impulse propagation is complete, unlike most batteries, recharging, or repolarisation, occurs very quickly through energy-dependent pumps (sodium/potassium ATPase) and the internal negative charge and ion differential is restored, ready for more activity.

Up to this point, a neurone appears to operate rather like an electrical cable, which is insulated externally with a substance called myelin and electrical impulses are conducted towards a target, which could be other neurones or a specialised junction between neurones and muscle. If the nervous system did operate like a standard electrical circuit, then one nerve would simply link up with another and the impulses would run along the system rather like one telephone line connected to another. However, this is not the case. When the neurone does meet another neurone it does not directly touch it; instead, a specialised junction, or 'synapse' is formed. Similarly, when a nerve meets a muscle fibre, they form a neuromuscular junction. From Figure 5.1, you can see that that nerve A at the top connects to the bottom nerve B through a synapse. Nerve A is termed 'pre-synaptic' and nerve B, 'post-synaptic'. The gap between the two nerves is termed the synaptic cleft. The process whereby information is conveyed so relatively slowly across a synapse used to strike me when I was a student, as rather like someone living on one side of a canal receiving a message by landline telephone. They then jump into a boat and row across the canal to the other side and find another landline to continue the call. Impulses from nerve A, which is 'pre-synaptic', cause calcium-controlled gates or pores open, allowing the release of a neurotransmitter, which travels across the synaptic cleft and binds to receptors which depolarise 'post-synaptic' nerve B. If enough neurotransmitter molecules bind enough receptors, nerve B is depolarised to the point that its sodium channels open and an impulse is triggered to the next neurone, or neuromuscular junction. From an evolutionary standpoint, this system has probably appeared to isolate neurones from each other so that information carriage can be fractionally delayed so it can be processed sequentially, rather like groups of microprocessors in an electrical appliance. It certainly works well enough in insects to make some of them extremely difficult to swat.

Hence, the neurotransmitter is the key chemical in nerve function and one of the most commonly employed neurotransmitters is acetylcholine (ACh). This chemical is made in the pre-synaptic area by an enzyme known as choline acetyltransferase (CHaT). During nerve impulse transmission, once ACh has finished binding

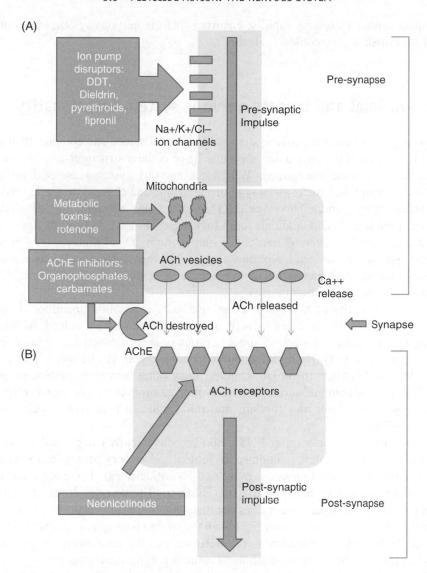

Figure 5.1 A synapse between neurones A and B: the various ion channels open to allow propagation of impulses along the body of neurone A towards the synapse, which then transduces the impulse into a neurotransmitter chemical movement, which eventually depolarises neurone B. The major insecticides impact pre-synaptically in neurone A (pyrethroids, fipronil, DDT), as well as in the neurone body affecting energy supplies (rotenone) as well as in the synapse, where they can inhibit acetylcholinesterase (AChE) to prolong the effect of ACh (OPs). Other agents hyperstimulate the ACh receptors (neonicotinoids).

to the post-synaptic nerve B receptors, it has to be removed, or it will continue to stimulate the receptors, like someone continuing to try to start a car with the ignition key after the engine has actually started. An enzyme has evolved to destroy ACh, called acetylcholinesterase (AChE). This enzyme thus switches off the neurotransmitter extremely rapidly, ensuring that the nervous system can control itself and modulate responses at all times.

5.6   Animal and insects nervous system commonality

Obviously a vertebrate nervous system is far more advanced and complex than that of an insect, but it operates using the same basic cellular structures and functional features, with some exceptions. Whilst all nervous systems use sodium and potassium channels, insects use a type of gated chloride channel controlled by the neurotransmitter γ-amino butyric acid (GABA) in their CNSs and muscles to stabilise neuronal activity and modulate inhibitory responses [32], and vertebrates do not use that system. However, all nervous systems require a very high capacity energy supply to power the various ion pumps as they push their substrates against concentration gradients. This means that neurones have large numbers of mitochondria, the main site of energy creation in cells.

The vast majority of nervous systems use ACh as a neurotransmitter at some point and insects rely on it extensively, in their CNS and PNSs; indeed, ACh neurotransmission can be mapped in insect nervous systems through measuring CHaT, as well as AChE [33]. If you have studied biology, you will be aware that aside from ACh and GABA, mammals employ many other neurotransmitters, such as noradrenaline, glutamate, serotonin and even histamine. However, many of us are not really aware of our own fundamental reliance on ACh in every aspect of the CNS and PNS.

As advanced vertebrates, our PNS could be conveniently categorised as having two main systems: somatic (voluntary movement and sensory perception) and autonomic (control of blood pressure, heart and breathing rates). There are important anatomical differences between the two systems. The somatic (from the Greek 'soma' or body) nervous system does not have junctions; this means that you could trace the neural supply from your big toe all the way to your spinal cord without any breaks. ACh is the neurotransmitter which operates the neuromuscular junctions between the somatic nerves and striated (voluntary movement) muscles.

The brain controls our involuntary activities through the autonomic nervous system which is divided into two sub-systems; one, the parasympathetic, controls smooth muscle (gut, vasculature, etc.) through cholinergic neuromuscular junctions and the other is the sympathetic, which operates smooth muscles using noradrenaline in its neuromuscular junctions. The difference between the somatic and autonomic systems is that the latter system has breaks in it, or groups of synapses called ganglia, which are operated with ACh. So even if a neuromuscular junction in the sympathetic system does not use ACh, if you trace any autonomic neurone from, say, the gut back to the brain, you will meet a cholinergic ganglion on the way. So the entire system relies comprehensively on ACh and therefore, if you recall the previous section, it also relies on AChE to manage the effects of ACh.

5.7 Major insecticide groups – ion pump disruptors

These include the organochlorine agent DDT and the pyrethroids, which lock open sodium pumps (Figure 5.1). This has the effect of preventing neurones from depolarising, which causes the nervous system to shut down, leading to insect paralysis. DDT is extremely cheap and effective, but resistance has grown rapidly and its persistence in the environment did enormous damage to ecosystems [34]. The pyrethroids are less controversial and probably the main insecticide of choice for domestic use at the time of writing. More than a thousand variants have been made, of which the most common are deltamethrin and permethrin. They are relatively low in toxicity to mammals, although there is increasing concern over their complex effects on mammalian cells as well as the immune system [35].

The GABA-gated chloride channels in insects as described in a section 5.6 are vulnerable to being blocked by the organochlorines lindane, endosulfan and dieldrin. This has an effect like jamming an engine throttle wide open and all inhibitory control of the insect's nervous system is lost, causing tremors, hyperexcitability, paralysis and death. However, these compounds are truly loathsome – they are persistent, non-selective and toxic to humans, both in terms of acute effects and also through their endocrine disruptor actions. Thankfully, they are in the process of being phased out [36], although these GABA-channels as a selective insecticidal target remained tempting for further insecticide development during the 1980s and 1990s. The result was a new class of inhibitors of these chloride channels known as the phenylpyrazoles. This includes picrotoxinin and fipronil; the latter agent will also inhibit other insect chloride channels, such as those operated by glutamate, down to nanomolar levels. Again, only insects use these channels and the combination of high potency and precise selectivity for insect life was intended to make fipronil safer than previous agents [37].

5.8 AChE inhibitors

The first effective inhibitors of AChE were the organophosphates (OPs), which were developed before World War II and are close structural relatives of the infamous 'nerve agent' OPs such as sarin, tabun, soman and VX. All OPs operate the same way and inactivation of AChE leaves ACh on its post-synaptic receptors for much longer than it would normally be left. Thus impulses would be conveyed postsynaptically in nerve B (Figure 5.1) which had not been transmitted through nerve A, which means that nerve B would then escape nerve A control. This would generate two huge problems for the organism. Firstly, nerve B would operate on its own and stimulate other nerves and muscles independently of the organism's will; and secondly, this rapid stimulation and repetitive firing would depolarise nerve B and any other nerves or muscles on the same circuit and eventually 'flatten' their battery, so to speak. This would mean that after only a few minutes, downstream of nerve A, the whole system would be unable to respond to a stimulus. The organism effectively loses control of itself rapidly and this is not practically reversible. There are other insecticides which block AChE and are toxic to mammals such as the carbamates carbaryl and bendiocarb [12]. They are reversible inhibitors of AChE, so in acute carbamate toxicity, patients are easier to treat compared with OP poisoning.

OPs are the cheapest and most ubiquitous AChE inhibitors and they vary enormously in potency. Some, such as fonofos, were so hideously and indiscriminately toxic that they were withdrawn. Indeed, its LD_{50} in rats is less than $20\,mg/kg$ (EPA fonofos), making it an EPA category I toxin. At the other end of the scale, malathion, which was often used to kill head lice prior to resistance problems, is around 50-fold less toxic than fonofos [38]. There are many other agents in category II that are known to be toxic to man, such as chlorpyrifos and diazinon. Attempts have been made to withdraw the more toxic and persistent agents from the market, although they remain extremely profitable to produce, so they continue to be manufactured and used worldwide in large quantities [39]. From a toxicological perspective, it is easy to recommend most strongly that all of them should be withdrawn, as they are acute and chronically neurotoxic and they also exert developmental toxicity on children and young adults [40]. In addition, they devastate wildlife and damage ecosystems. Users of these agents would defend them on the grounds that they protect crops in poor developing countries, safeguarding incomes and providing export-led foreign currency income. However, those that use them, particularly in developing countries, are usually not properly protected and there are alternative agents which are not as toxic, although admittedly these are more expensive. In terms of their human toxicity, it is accepted that they are acutely toxic to man. However, as we will see in the second case history in this chapter, their chronic impact on humans remains strongly disputed and this has cast a long shadow over cases of suspected OP chronic occupational injury.

5.9   Other major pesticides

The neonicotinoids appeared in the 1990s and were intended to circumvent resistance to other pre-synaptic agents, such as the ion channel inhibitors and the AChE inhibitors. Agents of this type, such as imidacloprid and acetamiprid, mimic the effect of nicotine, which stimulates post-synaptic receptors, hyperexciting the insect's nervous system, leading to paralysis and death (Figure 5.1). They are EPA-class II and III agents and they are so toxic to bees [41] that they were banned in the European Union for two years from December 2013 (Amendment to European Commission Regulation No 540/2011). These agents are acutely toxic to humans, with ingestion of as little as $40\,mL$ leading to hospitalisation with symptoms similar to that of nicotine poisoning [42, 43]. However, they are thought to be of low risk of chronic toxicity to mammals, mainly because they have a much greater affinity for insect nicotinic receptors compared with those of humans [44].

Among the other major insecticides used, several target cellular energy formation by the insect, where they disrupt either oxidative phosphorylation (tebufenpyrad, rotenone and chlorfenapyr) or ATP formation (diafenthiuron). These agents are usually acutely toxic to man, but much less is known of their chronic effects in regular users. However, it is notable that rotenone is now an established laboratory means of creating a Parkinson's disease-like effect in animal models [45]. Vast amounts of fungicides are also used in complex mixtures and their toxicity to man is still under-researched [46].

5.10 Case histories

As you have read, it is clear that all nervous systems have vulnerable points and pesticide designers and manufacturers have produced a vast array of agents aimed at attacking insect nervous systems. It is beyond question that most insecticides and several herbicides are extremely toxic if ingested in quantity by humans, which is not surprising due to the high amounts consumed in suicide bids, or during some accidental exposures. Writing a causation report when an agent has acutely poisoned an individual is straightforward, as there will be evidence of the amounts ingested, how this occurred, as well as symptoms and treatment details. There is plenty of clinical work in the literature available to cite which might support the evidence to link the agent with the effects in the victim.

However, what is much more difficult to approach is how to evaluate causation when exposure does not necessarily immediately lead to any reported symptoms, or perhaps only occasional symptoms. So the individual might work with an agent or agents for many years and not complain of problems, then some injury or health issue becomes gradually apparent which might curtail a working life. Without either a direct link to the agent in terms of symptoms and evidence of exposure or even very much literature to read and support the case, it can be quite a challenge to argue that a pesticide could be responsible for the health effects manifested. This is particularly difficult where the effects are neuropsychiatric, such as, for example, depression or cognitive impacts. These can be caused by a host of other factors which are hard to eliminate from the causation stream. There are yet other cases where an agent causes a long-term impact from a single exposure in an individual and there is little or nothing in the scientific literature to support that case either. These following cases do emphasise the value of the clinical and experimental literature precedents in mounting a causation argument and their power to confound or support any individual case.

5.11 Case history 2: Mrs L and fipronil toxicity

Mrs L sought professional veterinary advice about her dog's flea infestation and she was recommended to use a proprietary anti-flea spray known as 'Frontline™', which contains fipronil. This agent is still available and claims to kill fleas and ticks within 48 hours and is effective for up to five weeks. Mrs L read the product guidelines and she took the trouble to dress in improvised protective clothes, including wellington boots, a thick anorak, as well as stout rubber gloves and even a hat. Mrs L sprayed her pet in a well-ventilated and spacious area and she completed the task in approximately three minutes, using less than the recommended number of pumps related to the dog's weight. The dog was sprayed on only one occasion, yet within 20–30 minutes Mrs L in her statement reported experiencing several neurological symptoms, including numbness of the extremities, tingling sensations and tinnitus. She described the tinnitus as 'hissing noises' and reported a hearing deficit, although on medical examination her hearing was found to be normal. In addition, she stated that she suffered mental stress, fear and anxiety, as well as feeling the cold much more acutely than before the spraying episode. More than two years later, Mrs L was left with permanent symptoms, including 'numbness, tingling and bilateral tinnitus'. Her symptoms strongly impacted her working life, as she could not sit for long periods and had lost manual dexterity due to the neurological symptoms she was experiencing. Mrs L's tinnitus also impaired her appreciation of music and her relaxation time. Soon after the incident, she contacted a local Veterinary Hospital over whether there was any antidote or treatment and she was referred to the manufacturers. They responded at first, but after three weeks of intermittent dialogue, the manufacturers told her they would only respond to her doctor. Eventually a suitable practitioner was appointed and he diagnosed a 'chemical poisoning'. Mrs L also suspected that her pet had sustained a similar injury at the time of her injury, as it started to chew its feet, which was thought by a veterinary practitioner to be due to some form of numbness also. Mrs L had been in good health prior to her exposure to fipronil. She was examined by another doctor and I was sent his report to read and try to establish some causation.

Two medical reports were commissioned in total, which both indicated that Mrs L was suffering from tinnitus, as well as peripheral neuropathy, with 'glove and stocking' loss of light touch sensation in the hands and feet. The medical evaluations also examined and ruled out all conventional causes of peripheral neuropathy, based on a battery of clinical laboratory tests carried out on blood samples supplied by the claimant. The medical reports emphasised the impact of the neuropathy and tinnitus on Mrs L's life, in terms of her leisure time, musical interests as well as her ability to work. Further tests were recommended, such as audiology reports and nerve conduction velocity evaluations. One of the reports suggested that Mrs L had suffered CNS and PNS damage and both reports agreed that Mrs L's problems were most likely to have been caused by the fipronil exposure.

A report submitted by Dr M.D. Coleman written in response to the report of Dr X on the instructions of XXXX Solicitors concerning the case of Mrs L.

Instructions

Dr X's report on Mrs L indicates that she is suffering from a left peripheral vestibular lesion and I have been invited to comment on potential for fipronil to cause this pathology.

General fipronil-related toxicity

1. A report on the joint meeting of the FAO Panel of Experts on Pesticide Residues published in 1997 [47] states that 'Although fipronil is selectively toxic to insects, some of the toxicity of fipronil observed in mammals also appears to involve interference with the normal functioning of the GABA receptor.' This report also highlighted the persistence of fipronil-related material (half-lives recorded of hundreds of hours in rats) and the greater toxicity of a derivative of fipronil, desulfinyl fipronil, which is formed by exposure of the pesticide to sunlight. The human exposure which was deemed safe on a daily basis for fipronil was 0–0.0002 mg/kg body weight, while acceptable exposure to the desulfinyl derivative was 0.00003 mg/kg, which is 6.6 times lower than that of fipronil [47].

2. It is possible that the spray that Mrs L used may have had been exposed to enough light to form the desulfinyl variant of the pesticide. The report goes on to say: 'in summary, the toxicity of fipronil-desulfinyl is qualitatively similar to that of fipronil, but the dose–effect curve for neurotoxic effects appears to be steeper for fipronil-desulfinyl than for fipronil. Also, fipronil-desulfinyl appears to have a much greater tendency than fipronil to bind to sites in the chloride ion channel of the rat brain GABA receptor. This finding appears to be consistent with the greater toxicity, relative to fipronil, of fipronil-desulfinyl in the central nervous system of mammals' [47].

In addition, the report highlighted another study on rats which detected significant signs of neurotoxicity including 'irritability to touch' [47].

Possible fipronil-mediated audiovestibular damage

1. Fipronil is a relatively new insecticide and little human toxicity has been documented. To my knowledge, there are no existing reports that have investigated the effects of this agent on human audiovestibular physiology. However, it is possible to argue that fipronil is capable of causing damage in this area.

Mode of action of fipronil

1. Fipronil blocks receptors that are regulated by GABA, which is a major brain neurotransmitter. The receptors act like switches and control the movements of ions which operate neural function. Fipronil is known to block GABA-controlled chloride ion movement, which results in uncontrolled nervous system activity and death in the insect.

Vestibulo and reticulo-spinal neuronal systems

1. These systems are part of a reflex system which automatically compensates for changes in the body's position in space and time. For the system to operate optimally, input on body position from the semicircular canals in the inner ear and

visual information from the eyes must be processed almost instantly alongside other sensory systems (proprioreceptors in the neck) and translated into corrective movements in the body's musculature to maintain posture, balance and allow all the movements which are part of daily life.

2. Any interruption in the constant flow of information from the sensory areas (inner ears/eyes) to the rest of the brain will result in problems with balance/gait and posture. Dr X indicates that Mrs L's inner ear problems are leading to the effect that she feels she 'is moving continuously to the right side'.

GABA-mediated functions

1. GABA regulates many neural functions and recent research has indicated that in the chick and the rat [48, 49] the GABA-controlled receptors operate in the vestibular system. In the rat, inputs into the vestibular system were also GABA-ergic [48]. In the vestibular–oculomotor system, chemical antagonists of GABA abolished the functioning of these systems in rats [50].

Link with fipronil with audiovestibular toxicity

1. Overall, GABA-ergic transmission occurs in the vestibular systems across animal and bird species, so it is highly likely that this is the case in humans. As fipronil is a potent GABA antagonist, it is reasonable to suppose that it was capable of damaging Mrs L's audiovestibular system.

Summary

Overall, the known ability of fipronil to exert some aspects of its insect toxicity to mammalian systems suggests that it is capable of causing human toxicity. The presence of GABA-ergic receptors in the areas where Mrs L sustained damage suggests that the parent compound, a metabolite or a degradation derivative such as desulfinyl fipronil, was responsible for her symptoms and permanent impairment.

Yours faithfully,
Dr Michael D. Coleman

5.11.1 Case comment

At this point, the solicitor handling the case reviewed the claim with Counsel and sent me a number of questions to address, including a response from the manufacturers denying that fipronil was responsible in any way. The solicitor raised concerns about the droplet size which might have been created during the process of Mrs L's pet spraying, as well as asking my opinion on Mrs L's initial question about antidotes to her poisoning addressed to the Veterinary Clinic.

Addendum to a report submitted by Dr M.D. Coleman on the instructions of XXXX & Co. Solicitors concerning the case of Mrs L.

Dear Mrs Y,

There follows a reply to comments listed on your letter:

1. Droplet size governs where the agent will contact the respiratory or the gastrointestinal (GI) tract. Droplets/particles less than 10 μm will reach the deepest areas of the lungs, whilst large droplets will be trapped by the cilia (microscopic wafting hairs) on the bronchi and then transported to the stomach. The smaller particles/droplets of a substance could cause deep airway irritation/inflammation, whilst the larger particles would have more impact on the GI tract, from the stomach onwards. My feeling is that the droplet size is not really relevant in this case, as the agent is so lipophilic (oil soluble) and will be rapidly absorbed by either the lung or stomach. Neither site was listed in Mrs L's symptoms as far as I am aware. The speed of the symptom onset suggests a rapid entry of the agent into her blood.

2. Regarding their possible liability in this case, the manufacturers state (paragraph 1, page 2) that the product 'is a licensed medicinal product for veterinary use, which satisfies all the regulatory requirements with regard to safety and efficacy'. In the case of a drug which has caused a severe and untoward reaction in a patient, the manufacturer can claim that they satisfied the authorities that the product was safe. Consequently, they might feel that any claims/problems would be the responsibility of the regulatory authority. However, with drugs, the process of regulatory evaluation depends on full and frank disclosure of all necessary and relevant documentation on the safety of the product, such as animal and human trials of exposure.

   Effectively, drug companies were (and are) often aware of a particular possibility of a reaction in a certain number of patients based on results from their clinical trials. These data do not always reach the regulatory authorities, or are 'buried' in mounds of submitted documentation. I could find no published studies on the effects of this insecticide on humans, but animal data will be available and clues to a possible human response would be found there. At some point, an evaluation must have been made on the possible risks to humans of this product by the manufacturer or the manufacturer's parent company. If a full disclosure has not been made to the regulatory authority, then the liability should rest with the manufacturer, rather than the UK regulatory body.

   The second paragraph (page 2) contains a sweeping statement that there is 'no theoretical causal relationship between Frontline spray and your client's symptoms'. They do not attempt to qualify or explain the statement, nor have they any stated scientific credibility. Indeed, the statement sounds like wishful thinking on their part. I would have thought it clear to most laymen that an agent which disrupts insect nervous systems could have a similar effect on a human nervous system. Much publicity has been given to servicemen suffering from the alleged 'Gulf-War Syndrome' which has been partly ascribed to insecticide exposure.

As to their instructions for use (paragraph 3, page 2), it is impossible to comply with the 'do not breathe spray' instruction. How is this to be achieved, given that it has been conceded that the product could be used in a 'well-ventilated room'? Even in the open air, it is unlikely spray inhalation could be avoided. The 'do not breathe spray' implies that information on the possible human toxicity of this agent does exist, is available to the manufacturer and that the agent is toxic.

The company pointed out in their letter that Mrs L did not seek contemporaneous medical advice, that is, immediately, or as rapidly as possible. This was because she stated that she walked her dog after using the spray and experienced other symptoms as the day progressed, but did not seek medical advice until the next day. The company stated that because of this delay, there was no medical evidence to support the claim.

I cannot see how the urgency of the process of seeking medical advice affects the causality of the symptoms suffered by the patient. Patients are not often immediately fully aware of the causation and gravity of their symptoms. In any case, the peripheral neuropathy can be checked and validated by a physician (I assume that this has occurred).

3. I feel that a product such as fipronil should not be inhaled or contacted with bare skin at all. A filtered mask should be worn with gloves, the spraying should take place outdoors and the clothing used washed immediately (separately from other clothing). Unfortunately, the mask is not a legal requirement and the public do not have easy access to good quality filtered mask.

4. In cases of nerve agent toxicity, it is usually the case that the only protection that exists is pre-treatment with either a similar agent which blocks the effect on the nerves (hence it will also protect the insects) and such agents are also toxic. The use of such agents has been a suggested cause of 'Gulf-War Syndrome'. Once neural toxicity has occurred, there is little than can be done as neural cells repair themselves extremely slowly or sometimes not at all. Mrs L's symptoms might have improved since her exposure, but a point will be reached when there will probably be no more improvement.

Yours faithfully,
Dr Michael D. Coleman

5.11.2   Further case comment

Mrs L's experience with fipronil was only four years after the agent was first licensed and very little human data could be found at the time the reports were compiled. At the time of writing, now more than 13 years after she sustained her injury, it is apparent that fipronil is more toxic than was appreciated when it was first marketed. This is partly due to its sheer marketing success as more than 40% of US homes now use this agent in some form [51] so millions of individuals are exposed to fipronil daily. Although this agent has been extensively investigated for its toxicological effects, there remains relatively little work available on its human toxicity. A study which collated human case reports of injury with fipronil found that more than half involved women and about third of incidents were after residential spraying [52]. The authors stated that (pp. 740–741):

Consistent with the fact that the central nervous system is the primary target of fipronil, neurological symptoms were the most commonly observed health effects.

Having said this, the majority of problems were of low impact and were temporary, such as dizziness, headache, paresthesia, muscle problems and various cutaneous reactions like hives and rashes [52]. The individuals who suffered the most severe effects were pest control professionals, one of whom had a seizure, as well as dizziness and blurred vision. What is certainly the case is that the manufacturer's claims for the residual effects of the agent are justified. Four weeks after spraying, stroking a pet will result in transfer of fipronil to one's hands [53]. What is also interesting is that fipronil will cause toxicity to animals [54]. When the report was written, the main theme suggested that fipronil's GABA-mediated effects were responsible for her injury. Subsequent published research if anything has strengthened this hypothesis. However, now, as then, the problem in this case is not only the severity of her injury, but also its permanent impact on both her CNS and PNS. The author could find no similar case in the scientific and medical literature even at the time of writing, which mirrored Mrs L's symptoms. Even in clinical reports where significant overdoses had been taken, recoveries were complete and a fatal case was due to the subject consuming over 100 mL of insecticide [55]. However, a considerable number of reports have emerged which demonstrate the cellular toxicity of fipronil in neuronal and other *in vitro* cell models [52, 56]. The agent can cause cells to enter programmed cell death (apoptosis) and it damages mitochondrial function, causing similar effects to other insecticides such as rotenone. Fipronil also deranges neuronal cell development, as well as binding to human GABA receptors [52, 57]. Hence, it is possible that fipronil may have caused some form of programmed cell death in Mrs L's CNS and PNS. If this was the case, it could account for the lack of recovery over the 24 months post exposure. In the original report, the possibility that the fipronil used in Mrs L's spray was exposed to light and the more potent disulphinyl derivative formed in quantity was discussed; this again might have been an exacerbating factor. Overall, it is highly likely that Mrs L did suffer injury from fipronil and literature published over the last decade supports this contention, although the aetiology of her particular symptoms appear to be without precedent in the scientific literature.

The manufacturer's initial forthright rejection of the claim was very similar to that seen when an individual tries to claim on their travel insurance. Essentially, the position is 'go away, you have no chance'. Whilst this is somewhat distressing to the claimant, it is simply a common position adopted by the defendant that 'pulls up the drawbridge' and is intended to dissuade the faint hearted, so to speak. In many cases, such a flat denial will be successful in discouraging enough claimants to save a manufacturer a great deal of money. However, that initial statement by the manufacturer was not prepared by an individual with a scientific background, as they stated that there was no theoretical basis for Mrs L's symptoms, a position that was untenable at the time the report was written and is even more outrageous today.

However, it does appear that Mrs L was unusually sensitive to the effects of fipronil and had an atypical response. At the time I felt that she had a strong case, although I was not told of the final outcome. It is probable that the manufacturer may well have settled out of court. The toxicity of fipronil to humans has not dented its popularity or its profitability. However, given that around a third of the world's food is dependent on bees and only four billionths of a gramme of fipronil is lethal to an individual insect [56], perhaps fipronil's days may be numbered after all.

5.12 Case histories: OPs

The following two case histories illustrate the problems of writing causation reports in the sphere of OP pesticides. As stated earlier, there is no argument over the acute impact of these chemicals, but the issue of chronic health consequences is extremely complex. Not only is it difficult to argue that a health impact has emerged from chronic exposure without acute toxicity (so-called sub-threshold or sub-acute toxicity), but it is clear from reading the reports that many of the symptoms described are somewhat vague and could be ascribed to a variety of different causes, ranging from circulatory problems, arteriosclerosis, minor strokes or just some manifestations of a compromised immune system and normal aging. There are some parallels between exposure to solvents and OP effects and in both areas proving a causative link between a chemical and possible memory and personality deficits can also be difficult, as of course no matter how many times the individual's performance is measured, it is not possible to compare the results with their pre-occupational self. Performance in cognitive tests can be measured against population data, but again, this is not necessarily definitive. One of the major effects reported with OP exposure is depression, which is known to be extremely common and attributable to many causes.

Regarding causation reporting, it is important to document the level of exposure from the claimant's account and to try to identify which specific chemicals were involved, given the somewhat understandably sketchy descriptions supplied by the claimant. Whilst the claimant's statement is just one view, it is helpful to try to find evidence in the account which verifies the claimant's statement with regard to exposure in a way that they themselves might not necessarily link with the chemical. As the claimant is unlikely to be from a scientific or medical background, this can sometimes remove an element of bias in their account, although these days a few internet searches in the area of the chemicals involved by the claimant would provide plenty of symptomatic detail which could potentially bias an account. If the claimant does describe symptoms experienced at the time of use of the chemicals, it is useful to assess if these are commensurate with a considerable exposure. This could build up a picture of a history of exposure, which could perhaps be symptomless and sub-threshold, or alternatively, a series of considerable acute episodes, or perhaps even a combination of the two. The pattern of exposure might cast light on the severity and location of the symptoms, with reference to the available and relevant clinical literature.

In cases of OP occupational injury, claims have been submitted in such numbers that they have been the subject of a great deal of legal process and discussion over the past couple of decades. Towards the end of the 1990s, in some instances defendants, often the manufacturers, were facing multiple proceedings from many individuals and the causation issues, particularly with respect to neuropsychiatric problems, were extremely controversial and difficult to assess.

5.13 Case history 3: Mr M

Mr M had worked as a sheep farmer since leaving school and was exposed to sheep dipping with OP agents intermittently in the 1960s and then more regularly over 20 years from 1975. He had a very long medical history which was mainly concerned with influenza episodes, many of which were indicated to have been caused by infections. In the mid-1970s he suffered symptoms of unsteadiness on his feet and fainting. By the early 1990s, he developed persistent weakness in his lower limbs and episodes of severe vertigo, alongside numbness and speech slurring. In 1999, he suffered a collapse and was unresponsive for a period of a few seconds. Subsequent MRI scans and other investigations were unable to find a specific cause for these effects. His symptoms of chronic numbness persisted, along with tiredness and a feeling of general debilitation. He was found to be unable to work and had to take early retirement in his late fifties. An initial medical examination by a consultant neurologist resulted in a report which supported the contention that occupational exposure to the pesticides had contributed to Mr M's condition. A second medical examination and report could not find a clear link between the symptoms and OP poisoning. Legal proceedings were initiated against the manufacturers of two OP pesticides used by the claimant and I was asked to provide a causation report.

RE: An Expert Report prepared by Dr M.D. Coleman concerning the case of Mr M, born 1944.

Expert qualifications (as before)

Material instructions

I have been instructed to provide a basis for the biological plausibility of the injuries suffered by Mr M. I have also been asked to account for whether the individual symptoms suffered by Mr M can be linked to the products, that is, the OP insecticides that he used when he was a farmer/shepherd.

Introduction

To determine whether on the balance of probabilities the health impairment currently endured by Mr M is consistent with a form of toxicity, it is necessary to describe the nature of suspected toxin, the current scientific awareness of the biological effects of the agent and the potential for contamination. Finally, it will be necessary to evaluate the strength of the causality between exposure to the toxic agents and the symptoms currently demonstrated by Mr M.

OPs – mechanism of action

1. These agents ('nerve agents') were developed soon after the First World War and were intended to provide a more potent alternative to the various poison gases used in that conflict. They were designed to disrupt specific processes in the human nervous system to the point that it would catastrophically fail, leading to death within 10–15 minutes. The nervous systems of humans are usually classified as peripheral (the extremities) and central (the brain/spinal cord). The PNS can be further divided into the somatic (voluntary movement) and autonomic (control of heart rate, lungs, gut, etc.). The autonomic nervous system has junctions, or synapses, which rely on a chemical called ACh.

2. The somatic nervous system has junctions with muscle tissue (neuromuscular junction), some of which also use ACh. The main body of an autonomic nerve conducts an impulse, which is then conveyed by ACh across the synapse; the ACh is promptly removed by an enzyme called AChE. If the ACh is not removed by this enzyme, the system will quickly overstimulate the muscle it controls, effectively exhaust it and then cause a shutdown, or paralysis. OPs block AChE permanently and rapidly cause paralysis. ACh and AChE are also found in many other parts of the CNS.

OPs – acute symptoms

1. The first effects of OPs include hyperstimulation of the autonomic nervous system, leading to hypersalivation, production of mucus, lacrimation, as well as nausea and vomiting. Other effects include high blood pressure and a racing heart. Various muscles twitch violently until the intercostal muscles, which are essential for breathing, eventually become paralysed, leading to death.

2. There are a series of CNS effects that also occur, the milder ones include general weakness, drowsiness and lethargy, difficulty in concentrating, slurred speech, confusion and emotional lability. More severe CNS effects include convulsions, loss of consciousness and coma, leading to death [58].

3. Insects rely on AChE for many of the same functions that animals require, so they are vulnerable to the effects of OPs. Insecticide OPs are chemically similar to nerve agents, with minor structural changes which render them less toxic to animals than nerve agents such as sarin, soman and VX. However, they do exert their toxicity through the same mechanism as described earlier and, given sufficient exposure, will

cause similar symptoms. The number of accidental, suicidal or homicidal intoxications and fatalities with insecticide OPs exceeds 100,000 per year worldwide [58].

OPs – chronic effects

1. The chronic effects of OPs, whether from insecticide or nerve agent usage, are much more contentious than the acute effects. This is partly due to the exposure of farm workers to large numbers of other agrochemicals, which may also exert toxic effects over many years. In addition, farm workers can be exposed to diseases that have neurological effects, such as Lyme's disease. Although the acute effects of OPs are easy to account for, our incomplete understanding of the CNS contributes to the lack of clarity of the mechanisms of how OPs can cause long-term CNS disruption.

2. Regarding sheep dip, a condition known as 'sheep dipper flu' has been described, which has been regarded as a common, short-term consequence of exposure to OPs (Royal College of Physicians and Royal College of Psychiatrists, 1998), but there has been no comprehensive explanation on the detailed aetiology of this illness and how it is linked to sheep dip. However, studies on human cellular systems in the laboratory indicate considerable toxicity does occur after exposure to OPs such as diazinon [59].

3. The most commonly reported long-term OP-related deficits of the CNS include impaired vigilance, reduced concentration and information processing, psychomotor speed and memory capacity. In addition, depression, anxiety and irritability are also recorded [60, 61]. These effects can persist for more than 10 years after exposure ended [58]. Studies of workers in nerve agent factories have shown major deficits, which included permanently reduced vitality and decisiveness, neurovegetative disorders, such as cardiovascular, GI complaints, reduced libido and these individuals appeared to be 'pre-aged' [62].

4. Delayed neuropathies are common with OPs, to the point that standardised tests with sensitive avian models (hens) have been designed to test new insecticide agents. Intermediate syndromes are more controversial and it is unclear whether asymptomatic OP exposure does lead to any chronic effects. It does appear that repeated episodes of OP intoxication, whether mild or more serious, will lead to persistent CNS problems. These episodes may or may not have been recognised by the patient. More recent work has also suggested that the reason why some sheep dip OP insecticides are more toxic to some farmers rather than others can be explained by differences in their respective abilities to metabolise these agents [63].

Potential for contamination with OPs

1. It is well documented that guidelines for handling of OPs in their concentrated and dilute forms have been either adhered to with little enthusiasm or have been disregarded [58, 64]. The design of sheep dip equipment has also changed radically in recent years to prevent contamination of workers during the process of treating the

animals, which is almost guaranteed to lead to exposure of the operators to the agents. Animals often are required to be immersed in the dips for more than one minute and completely submerged for short periods [64].

2. Many sheep dip preparations are now designed to minimise handling to the point that the concentrate is simply put in a dissolvable bag into the trough; in previous years, there were ample opportunities for contamination with concentrate and diluted form. The concentrated forms are more than capable of entering the body through unprotected or denuded skin. In the process of sheep dipping, the dip can easily bypass the gloves and protective equipment due to the amount of thrashing about that a panicking animal may demonstrate.

3. Current estimates of toxic exposure to sheep dip are relatively low, around 1/1000 [64], although this may reflect improvements in dip apparatus design, the use of less toxic agents and more general awareness amongst the farming community of the potential toxicity of sheep dip chemicals and their consequent increased diligence in wearing protective equipment.

The link between OPs and Mr M's ill-health

1. Mr M used sheep dips which contained OPs from the late 1960s to the early 1990s. During this time, it is clear that the level of chronic contamination he endured was considerable, and on one occasion he fell into the dip himself. In the 1960s there was very little awareness of how chemicals could cause toxicity in most industries and the level of protective clothing worn was relatively low. General compliance with instructions for usage with toxic compounds was also poor compared with today. Mr M's medical records show a general pattern of 'flu-like' illnesses which began in the early 1970s and continued to the late 1980s. Although there are many viral causes of 'flu', OPs are strongly associated with this type of illness. The possible reason for this may be due to the direct effects of OPs on the autonomic nervous system, where increased secretions to mild parasympathetic stimulation may lead to irritation and consequent infection.

2. Some CNS-related symptoms ('head spinning' and 'giddy') were recorded by his doctor in 1974 (5/11) and 1975 (23/1) which bear some passing resemblance to his more recent 'funny turns' where he becomes unresponsive for several minutes at a time and which led to a traffic accident in 1992. The biological basis for these attacks, which were originally diagnosed as transient ischaemic attacks (TIA), is difficult to account for. The neurologist, in her comprehensive report, felt that these attacks did not conform to the TIA pattern seen in patients with atherosclerotic disease.

Possible biological basis of the 'funny turns'

1. Although OPs effectively destroy the AChE enzyme, the effects of partial inactivation of a neural system by these agents are poorly understood. There are a number of neurological conditions which are progressive in their disorganisation and eventual destruction of the CNS which have unknown causes, and repeated

investigations only uncover the consequences, rather than the mechanism of deterioration, such as motor neurone disease and multiple sclerosis.

2. Damage to groups of nerves that modulate other neural functions can cause general neurodegeneration and nerves can 'die back' from extremities. Perhaps it might be useful to determine if Mr M's condition has deteriorated since the previous bank of tests conducted by the neurologist. It is conceivable that exposure to OPs may have caused damage to the central control of the autonomic nervous system which leads to episodic periods of non-responsiveness. There may be some precedent for this in other neurological disorders of varying severity that occur with little warning due to known stimuli, such as epilepsy and migraines.

Specific OP agents encountered by Mr M

1. From Mr M's description of his sheep treatment activities, he dipped for blowflies and scab, among other parasites. 'Seraphos' was one of the agents to which he was exposed; the trivial chemical name for this agent is 'propetamphos'. Technical grade propetamphos is a yellowish, oily liquid at room temperature and is an OP insecticide designed to control cockroaches, flies, ants, ticks, moths, fleas and mosquitoes, where vector eradication is thought necessary to protect public health. It is also used in veterinary applications to combat parasites such as ticks, lice and mites in livestock. Commercial products include aerosols, emulsified concentrates, liquids and powders.

2. Obviously, no metabolic studies have directly dosed humans with this agent at levels likely to cause toxicity, and it has only recently been possible to track exposure to the agent by the use of a new method [65]. However, effects due to acute exposure to propetamphos will include those that occur with exposure to any other OP pesticide, including neurological and neuromuscular effects due to cholinesterase inhibition. Symptoms of acute exposure to OP or cholinesterase-inhibiting compounds such as propetamphos are commonly listed as: numbness, tingling sensations, incoordination, headache, dizziness, tremor, nausea, abdominal cramps, sweating, blurred vision, difficulty breathing or respiratory depression, and slow heartbeat [58].

3. The second agent to which he was exposed appears to be diazinon, which is found in some commonly used pesticide preparations branded as 'Coopers', such as the '4 in 1' dip and 'Di-Jet'. Diazinon is actually the commonest OP used in sheep dip in the United Kingdom. This compound is an organothiophosphate that displays similar toxicity profiles to OPs in general. The pure chemical is a colourless and practically odourless oil. Preparations used in agriculture and by exterminators contain 85–90% diazinon and appear as a pale to dark-brown liquid. A recent study on farmers has shown that this agent may be more toxic in some individuals due to genetic factors [66]. The compound is certainly very toxic to mammals [67].

Conclusions

Mr M reports impaired memory, irritability, apathy, as well as insomnia, fatigue, urinary problems and numbness in limbs and face. This is despite the observation that nerve conduction tests have not shown any peripheral deficits. These symptoms suggest that a pattern of CNS and autonomic nervous system damage may have been sustained. The neurologist has examined Mr M at length and conducted a number of recognised neuropsychological assessments on him. She has also evaluated other possible medical causes of the symptoms he describes and feels that she can eliminate them from the search for causality. The neurologist has observed that the pattern of deficits seen in Mr M is consistent with OP poisoning and I agree.

Schedule of symptoms

All OPs cause the same toxic effects, as the agents are all chemically similar. Their structural variations are linked with their stability, persistence, specificity and potency.

Described symptom	Link to OPs (e.g., diazinon/propetamphos)
Chronic 'flu-like' symptoms Over years of working life	Strongly linked with mild OP intoxication
Glove and stocking neuropathy, numbness of limbs	Linked to OP exposure, peripheral neural damage
Dizziness, slurred speech	Linked to OP exposure
Impaired memory, cognitive deficits	Linked to OP exposure
Anxiety, depression, irritability	Central effects which are seen with OP insomnia exposure, but could also be stress-related
'Funny turns' periods of non-responsiveness	Possibly linked to a CNS OP-neuropathy

Opinion

I feel that on the balance of probabilities, Mr M's symptoms are a result of many years exposure to insecticides found in sheep dip, primarily OP agents. As neural tissue usually does not regenerate or heal, it is unlikely that his condition will improve. Previous studies have shown those exposed to OPs as 'pre-aged', which also describes the general state of Mr M's health.

Michael D. Coleman, Ph.D.
Lecturer in Toxicology

5.13.1   Case comment

A few months after receiving my first report, further information was requested by counsel regarding the regular loss of consciousness Mr M reported and how this could be linked with OP exposure.

RE: An Addendum to an Expert Report prepared by Dr M.D. Coleman concerning the case of Mr M, born 1944.

Instructions

It has been requested that I comment on Mr M's 'episodes of absence' and to what extent these episodes may be attributable to occupational OP exposure.

The symptoms

1. Mr M first reported episodes that he terms 'queer turns' in 1987, where his head was described as 'spinning'. Through 1990, he suffered from weakness in his lower limbs and in December 1992 he had a severe attack when herding sheep and found himself in a ditch.

   His other symptoms were limb numbness, dizziness, slurred speech, loss of memory, anxiety, depression and insomnia. Another attack in 1999 caused his left arm to become numb, he could not speak, was confused and then suffered from vertigo, crashing his van in the process.

2. Since this attack, he has suffered a number of episodes of slurred speech, vertigo and right-sided neurological symptoms, which usually last 10 minutes or so. During these attacks he is unresponsive to stimuli.

3. Other symptoms include mood swings and emotional lability. Professor X (a second consultant neurologist) has described Mr M's attacks as almost 'catatonic' in nature.

   Although these episodic attacks resemble the effects of mild strokes, there has been no evidence that this was the case from a number of clinical investigations. So far, no diagnosis of these 'queer turns' has been made.

Link with OP exposure

1. I was unable to find any clinical reports in OP affected patients which matched Mr M's attacks, although it is possible to argue that these attacks are likely to be linked to OP exposure.

2. In my previous report, I described how generally Mr M's symptoms were compatible with long-term OP exposure. He also exhibits a number of characteristics of what is termed 'Chronic OP-Induced Neuropsychiatric Disorder (COPIND)'.

   This syndrome describes the chronic effects of OP exposure in terms of CNS symptoms: these include confusion, lethargy, anxiety, depression, fatigue and irritability. Indeed, chronic anxiety levels in commercial crop sprayers was significantly higher than that of farmers exposed to lower levels of OPs [61].

3. All these effects are caused by altered brain function, therefore it is reasonable to suggest that Mr M has suffered some degree of brain damage caused by exposure to OPs. Although there are other causes of the symptoms described earlier, so far, none have been identified by several clinical investigations.

4. Regarding Mr M's 'episodes', positron emission tomography (PET) scans have shown that brain blood flow can be adversely affected for years after exposure to OPs [68].

   It is possible, therefore, that Mr M may be suffering from a recurrent OP-mediated disorder of blood flow to a specific brain area, which leads to stroke-like symptoms, without the same diagnostic neural features of a typical stroke patient.

5. A study published in 1991 showed that problems with memory, visuomotor speeds, problem-solving, motor steadiness and dexterity as well as other neuropsychiatric problems resulted from OP exposure in agricultural workers [69].

6. Regarding Prof. X's belief that Mr M requires a neuropsychological assessment, including somatosensory and cognitive evoked potentials, I agree that this would be illuminating.

   It is highly likely that Mr M's impairments would be detected if he were to be tested psychometrically. However, this may well not throw any more light on the aetiology of his 'queer turns'.

Conclusion

I believe that Mr M is suffering from the effects of years of OP exposure and that he displays a pattern of CNS symptoms which conform to the presentation of other agricultural workers who have been similarly exposed.

Although there is no direct published precedent for his catatonic episodes, I believe that it is likely that these also are linked with his OP exposure.

Michael D. Coleman, Ph.D.
Lecturer in Toxicology

5.13.2 Further case comment

Approximately two months later, the defendants requested I responded to several specific questions regarding causation. My response follows.

RE: Mr M (claimant) and XXXX LIMITED (defendant).

RESPONSE TO QUESTIONS TO DR M.D. COLEMAN PURSUANT TO PART 35 OF THE CIVIL PROCEDURE RULES

Question 1: What are the comparative human toxicities of insecticide OP agents with nerve agents and could Dr Coleman furnish more detail on how this toxicity occurs with respect to the chemical structures of the agents.

OP insecticides and nerve agents are very similar and are in the same class of chemicals. The same core structure built around a phosphate group is seen in all the nerve agents and you can also see it in the structures of two OP insecticides shown in Figure 5.2. However, with insecticides, the organic groups (R1 and R2) tend to be bulkier, so the insecticides are less volatile and are also less potent in their binding effect on acetyl cholinesterase, compared with the nerve agents. Therefore, the insecticides are less toxic to humans than the nerve agents and the dose–response curve is consequently

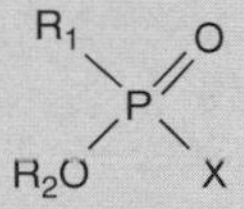

Nerve agents

Agent	X	R$_1$	R$_2$
Tabun (GA)	CN	N(CH$_3$)$_2$	C$_2$H$_5$
Sarin (GB)	F	CH$_3$	CH(CH$_3$)$_2$
Soman (GD)	F	CH$_3$	CH(CH$_3$)C(CH)$_3$
Cyclosarin (GF)	F	CH$_3$	C$_6$H$_{11}$.
VX	SCH$_2$CH$_2$N[CH(CH$_3$)$_2$]$_2$	CH$_3$	C$_2$H$_5$

Insecticides

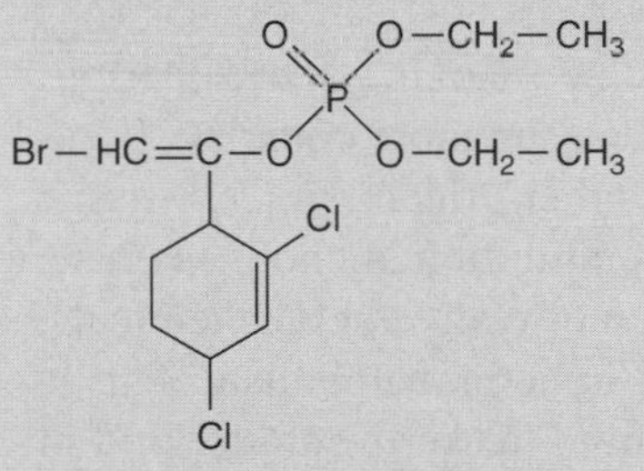

Bromfenvinfos

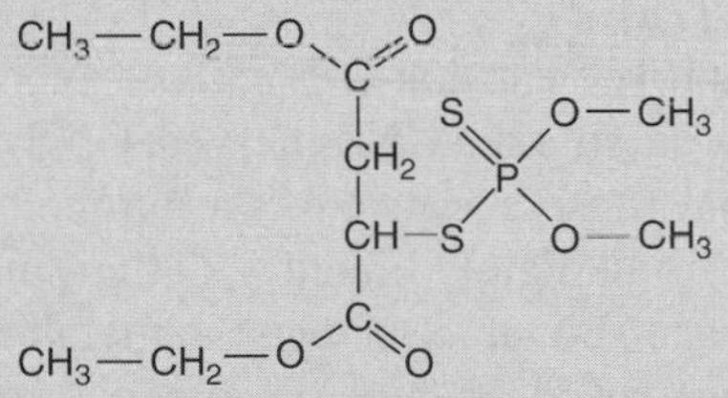

Malathion

Figure 5.2 This figure illustrates the basic structural similarity between the organophosphate 'nerve agents' and insecticides. Both types of agent possess the same organophosphate nucleus, differing in the size and the lipophilicity (oil solubility) of the side chains. These modifications are intended to make the insecticides less volatile and also less dangerous to mammals in comparison with the so-called nerve agents.

less steep with insecticides, despite their shared mode of action (described in the original report). The clinical effects of the insecticides are so close to the nerve agents that they are often used as laboratory models of nerve agent poisoning [70, 71]. Due to refinement in design of the compounds, nerve agents can be exceedingly toxic at low doses; in some cases, exposure of less than 300 microgrammes have caused serious illness [72]. Insecticides are at least an order of magnitude less toxic to humans, but more toxic to insects. However, it appears that the insecticides cause a more long-lasting disruption to cholinergic neural metabolism in the CNS compared with that of nerve agents [73], so it may be an oversimplification to directly compare dose/effect relationships. Exposure patterns may also differ, as repeated exposure to nerve agents is rare, while insecticides are more likely to be encountered at relatively low doses for long periods of time [74].

Question 2: How can OP agents cause CNS toxicity?

The CNS is obviously the most sophisticated system in living beings and the basic component, or neurone, is a complex entity in itself and its structure makes it uniquely vulnerable to toxicity compared with other tissues. The neurone is like a chemical electric cable, which possesses a myelin sheath, which means they are also insulated like an electric cable. There is a series of cells that maintain the myelin sheath and any long-term damage to these cells, for example, leads to loss of myelination and loss of neural conductivity and a condition such as multiple sclerosis develops. Toxins can also damage neurones and the cells can then 'die back' from an extremity, sometime after the insult; if the neurones survive they will be impaired, leading to a neuropathy [75].

Although it is clear that OPs cause a specific neurotoxic effect in peripheral (nerves outside the CNS) nerves, CNS effects are more complex. It has emerged that these agents exert a number of other effects on CNS tissue that are not immediately linked with their main inhibition of cholinesterase. OPs have been shown to change the metabolism of many neural chemicals, such as neuropeptides which have crucial roles in brain metabolism. This is rooted in the main design of OPs, which is to bind the serine amino acid in cholinesterase. This serine molecule is common to various systems which control these brain neuro-active substances, and this can also lead to the potentiation of the effects of some drugs, such as opiates, causing their effects to last a great deal longer [76, 77]. Studies on hens have indicated that delayed neuropathies due to OPs are complex and depend on age, species and chemical used. In hens dosed with protective agents, where they do not show any classic signs of OP poisoning, neuropathies still develop weeks after the end of agent dosage [78].

Stephens et al. [79] found long-term decrements in psychological test performances in sheep farmers who were exposed to OPs, often months after the last exposure. Another study with non-human primates showed that the animals showed a change in their EEG pattern which lasted 12 months after a very low non-toxic dose of a nerve agent [80]. With human neurodegenerative disease (Motor Neurone/Parkinson's/Alzheimers's diseases), we are often not aware whether these on-going conditions began from single or multiple exposure events, although it is better understood how they are sustained. In the case of chemical toxicity, such as with solvents and OPs, epidemiological studies establish patterns of exposure to specific agents, so a history of neurotoxicity can be examined during and after the exposure process. It is apparent that once CNS toxicity is sustained, individuals are often impaired for many years after the exposure ends or may continue to deteriorate [81–84].

Question 3: What is the link between Mr M's 'flu-like' symptoms and OP agents?

Some of the milder symptoms of OPs are caused by an initial overstimulation of the autonomic nervous system, which leads to increased lachrymation, nasal secretions, wheezing, increased bronchial mucous, increased sweating and cramps [85, 86], all of which are associated with 'flu-like' symptoms [87]. Mr M's records indicate that he suffered from repeated bouts of flu-like illnesses throughout the periods he was handling sheep dip agents.

Conclusion

There is a strong medical literature that supports the contention that OP exposure is capable of inducing long-term impact on human health. In view of Mr M's past documented exposure to OP agents in the course of his work in agriculture, I still feel that on the balance of probabilities, Mr M's current medical symptoms were caused by exposure to insecticides found in sheep dip, primarily OP agents.

Michael D. Coleman, Ph.D.

5.13.3   Final case comment

I was not informed of the outcome of this case, although I suspected that at the time it would not have proceeded. There were a number of reasons for this. The medical opinion was not unanimous that OP-exposure was to blame and in the detailed medical notes, more than one practitioner had noted that the claimant and his wife were adamant that he was suffering from OP-related problems and their response was quite vehement when they felt they were not being taken seriously enough. This may have led the medical examiners to feel that some of the claimant's symptoms were psychological in origin rather than directly linked with the OP agents. In addition, there were no detected abnormalities in Mr M's respiratory system. Moreover, the symptoms involving blackouts did not appear to have a strong enough link with previous reports of OP effects in the literature.

5.14   Case history 4: Mr N

This history was more complex, in that Mr N had worked as a farm labourer on mixed arable and livestock farms from around the age of 15, until he reached his late 50s. As most of us are aware, such work is extremely varied, requiring many different manual and technical skills. He spent many years operating machinery which distributed dozens of different agrochemicals on the land, including pesticides, fungicides and different crop yield enhancers of various types. He would also be required to treat the animals with several agents to combat different parasites. This involved regular pouring of chemical agents over cattle, as well as sheep dipping as described in the previous report. All these duties would involve handling the raw agent, then diluting it, followed by addition to distribution tanks where it would be sprayed on crops, or in the case of treating the animals, the chemicals would be mixed and then diluted in a trough for the dipping or pouring processes. He described how he would often become highly contaminated by the chemicals due to spray and dust inhalation, as well as splashing caused by the unpredictable reactions of the animals to the process. Over his working lifetime, he was exposed to such a range of different agents that it was surprising to me that he remembered so many of them, even if he often only recalled a slightly garbled version of the chemical. It is likely that his memory was aided by the seasonal and repetitive aspects to farming, where the same agents were used year after year at pretty much the same time. Mr N's experiences ranged over a 40-year sea-change in attitudes to Health and Safety and it is likely that his contamination with many of these agents would have been quite severe and repeated, particularly in the 1950s and 1960s, when the hazards of these chemicals were much less well known as they are now and there was no real control over usage of such products.

The handling solicitor wished me to determine from Mr N's occasionally hazy descriptions which agents were likely to have been involved. I was then to provide a causation contribution assessment for each agent in relation to his symptoms, which ranged from the psychiatric (depression and cognitive deficits) to the physical (severe urinary tract problems). This presented a complex research task where the most likely agent had to be identified from several possible chemicals in some cases. Some of the agents were probably innocuous, but an assessment had to be made as to whether the toxic entities could be reasonably linked with Mr N's health problems. At the time the report was commissioned, research on the impact of mixtures of agrochemicals on health was virtually unknown and even at the time of writing it is an emerging field, where some combinations of agents have been found to be significantly more toxic than the individual agents used alone [46]. Rather than pursue the manufacturers of the many agents to which he was exposed, Mr N took action against the legal representatives of the company that managed the farms he spent the most time working on.

An Expert Report prepared for the High Court by Dr M.D. Coleman concerning the case of Mr N, born 1943.

Expert qualifications (as previously described)

Material instructions

I have been instructed to advise as to whether on the balance of probabilities the signs and symptoms complained of by Mr N are capable of having been caused by his exposures to toxic substances as pleaded in the Particulars of Claim, that is, whether each such injury is biologically plausible.

1. Introduction
   To determine whether on the balance of probabilities the health impairment currently endured by Mr N is consistent with a form of occupational toxicity, it is necessary to describe the nature of suspected toxin, the current scientific awareness of the biological effects of the agent and the potential for contamination. Finally, it will be necessary to evaluate the strength of the causality between exposure to the toxic agents and the symptoms currently demonstrated by Mr N.

2. List of agrochemicals encountered by Mr N in his career
   This list has been drawn from Section 7.4 of the 'Particulars of Claim'; the spellings of the agents were presumably supplied by Mr N and contain a number of errors.
   Herbicides: 'banazolox' or 'Thiselaid/Falcon'; MCBA/CMPP, 'Multi-W' 'Pyremin' 'Gamacol (ICI)' 'Gestatop' 'Rounder' 'Isoproton'
   Insecticides: 'Matasystox-55' 'Folimat' 'Dursban' 'Sapecron' 'Aphox' 'Coopers Powerpack'
   'Youngs Sheep Dip' 'Rogor"E"', 'actellic-D', 'Cypomethrin'
   Molluscides: 'draza' and 'genesis'

3. Herbicides

3.1 'Banazolox' or 'Thiselaid/Falcon'
   This is actually 'benazolox', which is a mixture of two herbicides, benazolin and clopyralid. Benazolin is a systemic, growth-regulator herbicide, often used on oilseed rape crops. It is not very toxic to animals (acute oral LD_{50} for mice > 4000 mg/kg,

rats>6000 mg/kg) and is not irritating to the skin and eyes of rabbits. This agent is not thought to be toxic to humans. Clopyralid is a synthetic plant growth hormone and is highly persistent (up to 14 months in ground water). It is very irritating to the eyes (opaque cornea, inflamed iris, redness), and causes liver disturbances and urinary tract problems in experimental animals [88]. It is probably unlikely that either agent has contributed to Mr N's condition.

3.2 'MCBA/CMPP'

These spellings are incorrect and I can only guess at which agents are concerned. (4-Chloro-2-methylphenoxy)acetic acid is one possibility (MCPA), a phenoxyacetic herbicide. CDAA is another possible agent, an amide herbicide (2-chloro-N,N-di-2-propenylacetamide. MCPA acid is mildly toxic via ingestion yielding LD_{50} figures of 700 mg/kg to 1160 mg/kg in rats. Symptoms in humans from very high acute exposure could include slurred speech, twitching, jerking and spasms, drooling, low blood pressure and unconsciousness [88–90]. CDAA is linked with liver and kidney toxicity in animal studies and also displays potent skin irritant properties [91]. Although neither agent is without toxicity, these herbicides are unlikely to have led to the long-term effects on Mr N described in the 'Particulars of Claim'.

3.3 'Pyremin'

This is actually 5-amino-4-chloro-2-phenyl-3-(2H)-pyridazinone, known as 'pyrazon'. This agent controls broadleaf weeds. It is of a similar order of magnitude of toxicity to animals as banazolin and is not considered a skin irritant, nor is it believed to be toxic to humans [92].

3.4 'Rounder'

This is likely to be 'Roundup', an herbicide (glyphosate) that is still used in many domestic gardens. Aside from minor ocular irritation, there is no evidence that this agent is systemically toxic to animals or humans during normal application [93].

3.5 'Isoproton'

This is likely to be 'isoproturon' (3-(4-isopropylphenyl)-1,1-dimethylurea) a phenylurea herbicide, which is more toxic than banazolox (mentioned earlier), but around half as toxic to rats as MCPA(mentioned earlier) with an LD_{50} for rats of 1850 mg/kg. It can irritate the eyes and mucous membranes, but is not linked with severe human toxicity, nor is it thought to be neurotoxic in the long-term [88]. This agent is highly unlikely to have contributed to Mr K's condition.

3.6 'Multi-W', 'Gamacol (ICI)' 'Gestatop'

I was unable to find any information given these spellings, which may be incorrect or have been discontinued.

4. Insecticides

'Matasystox-55' 'Folimat' 'Rogor E' 'Dursban-4' 'Sapecron' 'Isoproton' 'Coopers Powerpack' 'Youngs Sheep Dip'; Considering the agents listed earlier, only 'Cypomethrin' and 'Aphox' (described later) are not OP insecticides or contain these agents.

4.1 OP insecticides

4.1.1 'Matasystox-55', or matasystox-R (*S*-[2-(ethylsulfinyl)ethyl] *O,O*-dimethyl-phosphorothioate), was used as a mitocide, although it was withdrawn in the United States in 1993.

4.1.2 'Folimat' (*O,O*-dimethyl *S*-methylcarbamoylmethyl phosphorothioate) is also known as 'omethoate' and is used as an acaricide.

4.1.3 'Rogor E' (2-dimethoxyphosphinothioylthio-*N*-methylacetamide), otherwise known as 'dimethoate', is an insecticide, nematicide and acaricide.

4.1.4 Dursban-4 (*O,O*-diethyl *O*-3,5,6-trichloro-2-pyridyl phosphorothioate), known as 'chlorpyriphos', is also an insecticide, nematicide and acaricide.

4.1.5 'Sapecron' (2-chloro-1-(2,4-dichlorophenyl)vinyl diethyl phosphate), known as 'chlorfenvinphos', is an insecticide and acaricide, which was withdrawn in the United States in 1991.

4.1.6 'Coopers Powerpack' (no longer available) was superceded by 'Coopers Ectoforce', the currently available Schering Plough product for OP control of sheep ectoparasites [94]. Both contain 'diazinon' (*O,O*-diethyl *O*-2-isopropyl-6-methylpyrimidin-4-yl phosphorothioate). Coopers Powerpack was originally supplied as a winter (40% diazinon only) and summer (40% diazinon plus 40% chlorfenvinphos) version. It is likely that 'Youngs Sheep Dip' also contained diazinon or a similar agent. Diazinon is the commonest sheep dip OP used in the United Kingdom.

4.1.7 Actellic-D contains pirimiphos-methyl(*O*-2-diethylamino-6-methylpyrimidin-4-yl *O,O*-dimethyl phosphorothioate), an acaricide and grain fumigant. This agent has been used in the United Kingdom since 1971 and was used in sufficient quantity to contaminate many wheat products (such as bread) to a significant degree.

4.2 OPs – mechanism of action

4.2.1 These agents ('nerve agents') were developed between the wars and were intended to provide a more potent alternative to the various poison gases used in the Great War. They were designed to disrupt specific processes in the human nervous system to the point that it would catastrophically fail, leading to death within 10–15 minutes.

4.2.2 The nervous systems of humans are usually classified as peripheral (the extremities; PNS) and central (the brain/spinal cord; CNS). The PNS can be further divided into the somatic (voluntary movement) and autonomic (control of heart rate, lungs and gut). The autonomic nervous system has junctions, or synapses, which rely on a chemical called ACh.

4.2.3 The somatic nervous system has junctions with muscle tissue (neuromuscular junction), some of which also use ACh. The main body of an autonomic nerve conducts an impulse, which is then conveyed by ACh across the synapse; the ACh is promptly removed by an enzyme called acetylcholinesterase (AChE).

4.2.4 If the ACh is not removed by this enzyme, the system will quickly overstimulate the muscle it controls, effectively exhaust it and then cause a shutdown, or paralysis. OPs block AChE permanently and rapidly cause paralysis. ACh and AChE are also found in many other parts of the CNS.

4.3 OPs – acute symptoms

4.3.1 The first effects of OPs include hyperstimulation of the autonomic nervous system, leading to hypersalivation, production of mucus, lacrimation, as well as nausea and vomiting. In addition, numbness, tingling sensations, incoordination, headache, dizziness, tremor, nausea, abdominal cramps, sweating, blurred vision, difficulty breathing or respiratory depression, and slow heartbeat can occur. Other effects can include high blood pressure and a racing heart. Various muscles twitch violently until the intercostal muscles, which are essential for breathing, eventually become paralysed, leading to death [90].

4.3.2 There are a series of CNS effects that also occur; the milder ones include general weakness, drowsiness, lethargy, as well as difficulty in concentrating, slurred speech, confusion and emotional lability. More severe CNS effects include convulsions, loss of consciousness and coma, leading to death [58].

4.4 OPs – insecticides and nerve agents

4.4.1 Insects rely on AChE for many of the same functions that animals require, so they are vulnerable to the effects of OPs. Insecticides and nerve agents are very similar and are in the same class of chemicals. The same core structure built around a phosphate group is seen in all the nerve agents and it is also apparent in the structures of all OP insecticides.

4.4.2 OP insecticides are less potent in their binding effect on acetyl cholinesterase compared with the nerve agents. Therefore, the insecticides are less toxic to humans than the nerve agents and the dose–response curve is consequently less steep with insecticides, despite their shared mode of action.

4.4.3 The clinical effects of the insecticides are so close to the nerve agents that they are often used as laboratory models of nerve agent poisoning [70, 71]. Due to refinement in design of the compounds, nerve agents can be exceedingly toxic at low doses; in some cases, exposure of less than 300 μm (300 millionths of a gramme) have caused serious illness [72].

4.4.4 Insecticides are at least an order of magnitude less toxic to humans, compared with insects. However, it appears that the insecticides cause a more long-lasting disruption to cholinergic neural metabolism in the CNS compared with that of nerve agents [73].

4.4.5 Exposure patterns may also differ, as repeated exposure to nerve agents is rare, while insecticides are more likely to be encountered at relatively low doses for long periods of time [74, 79]. The number of accidental, suicidal or homicidal intoxications and fatalities with insecticide OPs exceeds 100,000 per year worldwide [58].

4.5 OP CNS – chronic effects – range of opinion

4.5.1 The chronic effects of OPs, whether from insecticide or nerve agent usage, are much more contentious than the acute effects. The report produced by the Committee on Toxicity (COT) in 1999 addressed this situation in detail and reviewed the leading scientific studies carried out in agricultural workers in various countries [95]. The Committee felt that the limitations in much of current research meant that it did not support the contention that OPs cause long-term cognitive disorders, although they felt that 'the possibility that it (exposure to OPs) leads to neuropsychological disorders in a small sub-group of individuals cannot be excluded'.

It is often the case with human occupational exposure to toxins that the lack of controlled conditions seen in, say an experimental animal trial, means that there are too many confounding factors to strongly associate human health decrements with toxic exposure. The COT report drew attention to the defects in some studies on individuals who had been acutely exposed to high levels of OP insecticides [96] such as the lack of data on the degree of exposure to the OP involved and the variability of the impairments shown [95].

In addition, farm workers are also exposed to large numbers of other agrochemicals, as seen with Mr N, which may or may not also exert toxic effects over many years. Farm workers can also be infected with diseases that have neurological effects, such as Lyme's disease. There are other difficulties in conducting scientific determinations of human toxicity, such as the recruiting of sufficient numbers of individuals to make the study statistically valid. The COT report highlights a potential major problem with studying subtle cognitive adverse effects, where the individuals' prior conviction that they are already 'damaged' by the OPs could influence the testing procedures, leading to the recording of greater deficits than those that actually exist [95].

4.5.2 Although the acute effects of OPs are easy to account for, our incomplete understanding of the CNS contributes to the lack of clarity of the mechanisms of how OPs could cause long-term CNS disruption. This gives rise to a second problem described by the COT report, the lack of specific proven mechanisms for chronic OP CNS neurotoxicity [95].

4.6 OPs – CNS chronic effects

4.6.1 The CNS is obviously the most sophisticated system in living beings and the basic component, or neurone, is a complex entity in itself and its structure makes it more vulnerable to toxicity compared with other tissues.

4.6.2 The neurone is like a chemical electric cable, which possesses a myelin sheath, that acts to insulate it like an electric cable. There are cells that maintain the myelin sheath and any long-term damage to these cells, for example, leads to loss of myelination and neural conductivity and a neurodegenerative condition such as multiple sclerosis.

4.6.3   Toxins can also damage neurones causing them to 'die back' from an extremity, perhaps months later; if the neurones survive they will be impaired, leading to a neuropathy [75].

4.6.4   Although it is clear that OPs cause a specific neurotoxic effect in peripheral (nerves outside the CNS) nerves, CNS effects may be governed by other actions of OPs on CNS tissue and enzymes that are not immediately linked with their main inhibition of AChE.

4.6.5   OPs have been shown to change the metabolism of many neural chemicals, such as neuropeptides, which have crucial roles in brain metabolism. This is rooted in the main chemical function of OPs, which is to bind the serine amino acid in AChE. This serine group appears in many CNS enzyme systems and inhibition of serine groups can alter the effects of some drugs, such as opiates, considerably extending their duration of action [76]. Another mechanism is centred on 'neuropathy target esterase' or NTE [97]. The COT report listed at least four other possible mechanisms whereby OPs could damage the CNS based on their known chemical interactions with human neural tissue, although again, none have been conclusively identified [94].

4.6.6   Studies on hens have indicated that delayed neuropathies due to OPs are complex and depend on age, species and chemical used. In hens dosed with protective agents, eliminate the appearance of OP poisoning, neuropathies still develop weeks after the end of OP dosage [78]. In a number of countries, the hen model is used to detect delayed neuropathies caused by new insecticide agents.

4.6.7   A study with non-human primates showed that the animals showed a change in their EEG pattern which lasted 12 months after a very low non-toxic dose of a nerve agent [80].

4.6.8   The most commonly reported long-term OP-related deficits of the CNS in humans include impaired vigilance, reduced concentration, information processing, psychomotor speed and memory capacity. In addition, depression, anxiety and irritability are also recorded [60, 95, 98]. OP exposure has also long been linked with chemical sensitivity [99, 100]. These symptoms can persist for more than 10 years after exposure ends [58].

4.6.9   Studies of workers in nerve agent factories have shown major deficits, which included permanently reduced vitality and decisiveness, neurovegetative disorders, such as cardiovascular, GI complaints, reduced libido and these individuals appeared to be 'pre-aged', that is, displaying illnesses more usually associated with much older people [62]. One report [79] found long-term decrements in psychological test performances in sheep farmers who were exposed to OPs, often months after the last exposure.

4.6.10   Intermediate syndromes are more controversial and it is unproven whether asymptomatic OP exposure does lead to any chronic effects. A recent study on farmers who showed no acute illness related to long-term use of OPs showed only subtle exposure-dependent changes in neuropsychological performance, such as significant reductions in reaction times [101]. However, all the human studies carried out in workers exposed to OPs during the course of their work suffer from the limitations described in Section 4.5.1. However, it does appear that repeated episodes of OP intoxication, whether mild or more serious, can lead to persistent CNS problems; these episodes may or may not have been attributed to OP exposure recognised by the patient [96]. More recent work has also suggested that the reason why some sheep dip OP insecticides (such as diazinon) are more toxic to some farmers rather than others could be linked with differences in their respective abilities to metabolise these agents, although this type of investigation is in its infancy [63, 66].

4.7 Diazinon – exacerbating effects

4.7.1 The major OP that Mr N handled was diazinon in sheep dip. Improvements in the manufacture of this chemical since 1979 have significantly reduced the content of highly toxic impurities, such as tetraethyl-pyrophosphate (TEPP). As a result of these progressive improvements, the acute oral LD_{50} of technical grade diazinon has increased from 250 mg/kg to 1250 mg/kg in the rat. TEPP is also an OP [102] but it is much more toxic than other OP insecticides and has been fatal in man at doses of less than 25 mg [103]. It is apparent that Mr N used diazinon extensively up to 1979, when it was contaminated with TEPP; even without TEPP as a contaminant, diazinon remains a highly toxic agent to animal and human cells [59, 67].

4.8 Phenols – exacerbating effects

4.8.1 Phenolic agents, such as cresol/cresylic acid and o- and p-cresols were added to sheep dips prior to the early 1990s, primarily to prevent bacterial contamination and farmers believed that they would make the sheep 'smell right'. It is now clear that these agents were quite toxic in their own right. Animal studies have reported effects on the blood, liver, kidneys and CNS, and reduced body weight, from oral and inhalation exposure to mixed cresols. Several animal studies suggest that o-cresol, m-cresol and p-cresol may act as tumour promoters [103]. The pesticide manufacturers were unwilling to invest in detailed toxicity testing of these agents and the phenols were withdrawn from all sheep dips and cattle treatments by the end of 1993. It is possible that these agents may have exacerbated Mr N's CNS-related symptoms.

4.9 OP CNS toxicity – summary

Although it is proven that OP insecticides are acutely toxic, it is not proven to the satisfaction of a UK government advisor body such as the COT that they lead to chronic CNS impairment. COT acknowledged that it received many submissions from individuals who believed that OPs had impaired their health and it also recognised the severe degree of debilitation suffered. However, as humans cannot be included in studies which knowingly, under controlled conditions, expose them to varying levels of OP agents over many years, it is impossible to say when enough scientific studies might emerge which convince government advisory bodies that OPs can cause chronic neurological impairment. Paradoxically, with modern UK safety standards, better awareness of these agents' toxicity and the presence of fewer toxic impurities, it will become more difficult in the future to prove that OP exposure can lead to chronic CNS impairment. In my opinion, although absolute proof that OPs cause CNS impairment is lacking, on the balance of probabilities, it is toxicologically plausible to link such easily absorbed, reactive and neurotoxic chemical entities such as OPs with CNS-related illnesses in some individuals.

5. Molluscides and non-OP insecticides

5.1 'Aphox' 'draza' and 'genesis'
All three agents are carbamate insecticides and molluscides. They act in a similar way to OP agents, but with an important difference. Rather than irreversibly bind to the AChE enzyme, they carbamylate the AChE active site in a similar way to the drug neostigmine. This chemical bond is reversible (albeit very slowly), but this means that these agents show similar acute effects to OP insecticides, but recovery occurs relatively quickly. 'Aphox' (2-dimethylamino-5,6-dimethylpyrimidin-4-yl dimethylcarbamate) is also known as pirimicarb. 'Draza' slug pellets contain 3% methiocarb (4-methylthio-3,5-xylyl methylcarbamate) and 'Genesis' slug pellets contain 4% thiodicarb (7,9,13-tetramethyl-5,11-dioxa-2,8,14-trithia-4,7,9,12-tetra-azapentadeca-3,12-diene-6,10-dione).

It is believed that they will demonstrate additive effects when exposure occurs in the presence of OP insecticides, but by themselves they are not usually associated with such persistent deficits as OPs [95]. It is probable that exposure to these agents may have added to the effects of concurrently used OPs during the course of Mr N's farm work.

5.2 'Cypomethrin' V
Should be 'Cypermethrin', an insect peripheral neurotoxin, which is part of the class of 'alpha-cyano pyrethroids'. Chemically, it is defined as alpha-cyano-3-phenoxy-benzyl ester of the dichloro analogue of chrysanthemic acid, 2,2-dimethyl-3-(2,2-dichlorovinyl) cyclopropanecarboxylic acid. Although they act to disrupt neural function in insects, there is no evidence that they are systemically toxic to man, or interact with DNA [104], other than occasional effects on skin sensation, known as paraesthesia; poor absorption across skin means poisonings are very rare [105]. Although this agent is classified in the United States as moderately toxic, Mr K's symptom profile suggests that the probability that cypermethrin has contributed to his impairment is likely to be low.

6. Potential for contamination with OPs and similar agents

6.1 It is a requirement that animals should be immersed in the dips for more than one minute and completely submerged for short periods [64]. Many sheep dip preparations are now designed to minimise handling to the point that the concentrate is simply put in a dissolvable bag into the trough [94]; in previous years, there were more opportunities for contamination during the process of handling the concentrate and diluted form. The concentrates of OP agents included various toxic additives (as described earlier) and OP mixtures, often at up to 80% weight of OP by volume of solvent. Due to the lack of a sealed tractor cab system, Mr N's crop spraying activities also led to high contact with insecticide/

molluscide spray/dust, with ample opportunity to breathe the spray/dust and absorb the OP and carbamate agents.

6.2   Enormous amounts of research time and money have been spent to make OP agents absorbable by insects, so consequently an important route of insecticide/herbicide contamination is through the skin [106] and many insecticides contain detergents and other additives that greatly increase their ability to enter human skin; indeed, the choice of protective wear is crucial to avoid contamination [107].

6.3   In the process of sheep dipping, the dip can easily bypass the gloves and protective equipment due to the amount of thrashing about that a panicking animal may demonstrate. As Mr N comments, the sheep remember the previous dipping experience and are less cooperative as a consequence. Current estimates of acute toxic exposure to sheep dip are relatively low, around 1/1000 [64], and this reflects improvements in dip apparatus design, the use of less toxic agents, lack of contact with the insecticide concentrate and more general awareness amongst the farming community of the potential toxicity of sheep dip chemicals. This has also led to increased diligence in the wearing of protective equipment.

7.   Plausibility of the link between OPs and Mr N's ill-health

7.1   Opportunities for exposure
Mr N used sheep dips containing OPs from the 1960s to the end of the 1990s. During this time, it is clear that the level of chronic contamination he endured was considerable (up to 1500 sheep dipped annually at least once with mixtures of OP agents). This was compounded by his exposure to OPs in crop spraying while working in an unsealed tractor cab. Mr N was exposed to at least eight different OP insecticides for over 35 years. There were opportunities for the agents to enter his body by inhalation (Actellic-D during fumigation; Metasystox-R during crop spraying) as well as contact through his skin (diazinon, etc.) during the dipping processes.

7.2   Alcohol intolerance and OP exposure
I am unaware of any scientific literature that describes those exposed to OP agents developing a permanent intolerance to ethanol consumption, although it is known that OPs are sufficiently reactive to damage drug metabolising enzymes in the liver [95]. Indeed, it is possible to forward a more detailed explanation of this effect as it occurred in Mr N, based on recent research into OP metabolism in the human liver. Removal of sulphur from diazinon and its related OP agents occurs during the human liver metabolism [108]. Sulphur-related agents are potent inhibitors of one of the major liver enzymes which metabolise ethanol [109]. Indeed, a sulphur-containing drug, 'Antabuse', is employed to assist in the recovery of alcoholics [110]. If the patient drinks alcohol when taking Antabuse, they become violently sick in the same pattern that Mr N demonstrated. It is possible that Mr N's intake of OP-related agents was sufficiently high to interfere with the removal of ethanol from his blood, leading to the 'flu-like illness' he described after drinking lager. Mr N's intolerance to alcohol provides circumstantial evidence supporting the idea that OPs entered his body in sufficient amounts to affect his metabolism.

8. Schedule of symptoms: Links with chemical exposure
   The following section describes Mr N's main symptoms (as described in Particulars of Claim, section 16.2) and suggests which agrochemicals may be plausibly linked with the development of the conditions.

Symptoms	Cognitive impairment/psychomotor speed (memory and verbal fluency impairments)
Agents	'Matasystox-55' 'Folimat' 'Dursban' 'Sapecron' 'Coopers Powerpack' and
	'Youngs Sheep Dip' (diazinon) 'Rogor E', 'actellic-D', 'draza' and 'genesis'
Symptom	Depression
Agents	'Matasystox-55' 'Folimat' 'Dursban' 'Sapecron' 'Coopers Powerpack' and
	'Youngs Sheep Dip' (diazinon) 'Rogor E', 'actellic-D', 'draza' and 'genesis'
Symptom	Dizziness
Agents	'Matasystox-55' 'Folimat' 'Dursban' 'Sapecron' 'Coopers Powerpack' and
	'Youngs Sheep Dip' (diazinon) 'Rogor E', 'actellic-D', 'draza' and 'genesis'
Symptom	Chronic fatigue (lassitude/tiredness)
Agents	'Matasystox-55' 'Folimat' 'Dursban' 'Sapecron' 'Coopers Powerpack' and
	'Youngs Sheep Dip' (diazinon) 'Rogor E', 'actellic-D', 'draza' and 'genesis'
Symptom	Multiple chemical sensitivity
Agents	'Matasystox-55' 'Folimat' 'Dursban' 'Sapecron' 'Coopers Powerpack' and
	'Youngs Sheep Dip' (diazinon) 'Rogor E', 'actellic-D'
Symptom	Stiffness/muscle pain
Agents	It is difficult to directly ascribe a chemical causality for such non-specific symptoms, which may have a large number of possible causes

Opinion

I feel that on the balance of probabilities, it is plausible that Mr N's symptoms are a result of many years exposure to insecticides found in sheep dip and crop sprays, primarily OP agents. Of the other agrochemicals that he has encountered, it is possible that only the carbamate insecticides and molluscides significantly added to the burden of his illness.

Michael D. Coleman, Ph.D.
Lecturer in Toxicology

5.14.1   Case comment

When the first draft of this report was supplied to Mr N's legal team, it was reviewed by an expert in the field of OP litigation who criticised it heavily for failing to pay sufficient heed to the 1999 COT Report on OPs. This was a legitimate criticism, partly because the first draft did not fully describe the range of opinion, which is a major failing in a causation report. The expert used the phrase 'knockout blow' to describe the effect of the COT report on future claims of occupational OP-mediated damage. This is because it was a product of a joint working party of experts, who had taken the time to review all the available clinical literature, therefore, it carried much more significant scientific weight and credibility compared with any review, single report, or indeed anything I could write. Essentially, the expert implied that a copy of this COT report would be contained in the proverbial wall mounted '*In case of litigation break glass*' unit in the office of every OP pesticide manufacturer and supplier. Regarding the impact of the COT report, with any government working party, it is important to examine their precise remit. COT was asked to (page 2 of the report):

> …'advise on whether prolonged or repeated low-level exposure to OPs, or acute exposure at a dose lower than causes overt toxicity, can cause chronic ill health.'

It is clear from that statement that their remit does **not** include examining evidence as to the credibility of cases of acute poisoning by OP agents and their neuropsychiatric sequelae. So I think that the COT report is not a 'knockout blow' to all litigation, but rather it 'raised the bar' for claims, making it difficult for an individual to mount a successful case, who could not show that they had suffered from acute bout of OP poisoning which led to medically certified impact, long-term or otherwise.

Assuming a given claimant did not suffer an acute poisoning episode, the mainstays of their case over OP-mediated health problems would be establishing the degree of exposure, the biological plausibility and finally the citation epidemiological studies which supported the impact of these toxins on health. Regarding exposure, the COT report effectively undermined perceptions of how much exposure to OPs claimants really may have had and how much of the agents might have entered their systems. For instance, the COT report cited literature that did not support the idea that sheep dipping led to any significant contamination through inhalation and that being splashed with the dip (not the concentrate) did not correlate with increased urinary excretion of the metabolites of OP agents, so there was no 'spike' in measured metabolites which coincided with the increased exposure. In addition, they cited studies where sheep dipping did not significantly affect erythrocytic cholinesterase activity, again undermining perceptions of the level of exposure and entry into the body of the OP agents. The working party also did not even accept that 'dippers flu' was related to OP agents. The COT reviewed literature related to NTE as well as other esterase enzymes and they worked on the basis that if a particular effect is not seen after acute exposure, then it is not very plausible that the effect would be seen in an individual whose exposure was much lower. Through citing other studies, COT reported that the biological plausibility that OP agents could cause neuropsychiatric illness was not strong as the clinical evidence available was not convincing. Indeed, they described several manifest defects which undermined the clinical credibility of many studies. These problems included small study sizes and various biases, such as the participation in studies of individuals who were already convinced that they had been damaged by OP agents.

My own perspective when I wrote my report was that OP agents were a plausible cause of long-term neuropsychiatric effects, but in the face of what was effectively government opinion to the contrary, neither counsel nor a court would be likely to uphold my opinion over that of the expert group. However, as with any medical and scientific field, more research work is published continually and such evidence may either support or challenge current perceptions. Whilst the COT report was published in 1999, within three years a report had emerged that stated:

'The weight of current evidence is therefore very much in favour of the notion that chronic low-level exposure to OP produces neurotoxicity. Criticisms levelled against this notion are unfounded and probably misconceived' [111].

The OP agents were intended to block AChE and it has been known for many years that other crucial esterases found in the CNS, such as NTE, can also be blocked by these agents and may be linked with the central effects. However, over the last decade, it has become clearer that OP agents can impact a much wider range of enzyme systems that was previously realised. These chemicals can damage many basic neuronal functions, such as energy metabolism at the mitochondrial level, as well as specific processes vital to neuronal health, such as axonal transport; in addition, they generate oxidative stresses in neurones [112]. It now appears to be more widely accepted that there is a basis to neuropsychiatric OP-related health decrement and that acute symptomatic episodes are not necessary to cause these problems [113]. Indeed, as clinical research progresses, it is probable that the balance of opinion in the future will be less hostile towards sub-acute, OP-induced injury due to chronic exposure.

References

1. Michigan Technological University. 2012 October 12. Spotting a trend in the genes: three genes that cause cancer and disease in humans also 'paint' spots on butts of fruit flies. *ScienceDaily*. http://www.sciencedaily.com/releases/2012/10/121012143746.htm (accessed on November 15, 2013).
2. Greenspan RJ, Dierick HA. 'Am not I a fly like thee?' From genes in fruit flies to behaviour in humans. Hum Mol Genet, 13, R267–R273, 2004.
3. Reiter LT et al. A systematic analysis of human disease-associated gene sequences in *Drosophila melanogaster*. Genome Res 11, 1114–1125, 2001.
4. Gill RJ et al. Combined pesticide exposure severely affects individual- and colony-level traits in bees. Nature 491, 105-U119, 2012.

5. Agbohessi PT et al. Acute toxicity of agricultural pesticides to embryo-larval and juvenile African catfish *Clarias gariepinus*. Arch Environ Contam Toxicol 64, 692–700, 2013.

6. Watts, M. 2013. Paraquat. http://wssroc.agron.ntu.edu.tw/note/Paraquat.pdf (accessed on November 11, 2013).

7. Dodge AD, Harris N. The mode of action of paraquat and diquat. Biochem J. 118(3), 43P–44P, 1970.

8. Hsieh YW et al. Paraquat poisoning in pediatric patients. Pediatr Emerg Care 29, 487–491, 2013.

9. Routt-Reigart J, Roberts, JR. 1999. Recognition and Management of Pesticide Poisonings, 6th edition. United States Environmental Protection Agency (EPA) publication number: 735K13001, Washington, DC, 2013. http://www2.epa.gov/pesticide-worker-safety (accessed on November 15, 2013).

10. Kim J et al. Depressive symptoms and severity of acute occupational pesticide poisoning among male farmers. Occup Env Med 70, 303–309, 2013.

11. Nishijo M et al. Impact of perinatal dioxin exposure on infant growth: a cross-sectional and longitudinal studies in dioxin-contaminated areas in Vietnam. PLoS One 7(Jul 16), 2012.

12. Committee to Review the Health Effects in Vietnam Veterans of Exposure to Herbicides. 2004. Veterans and Agent Orange. National Academies Press, Washington, DC. www.nap.edu/catalog/11242.html#orgs (accessed on November 11, 2013).

13. Fishel F et al. 2013. Herbicides: How Toxic are They? http://edis.ifas.ufl.edu/pdffiles/PI/PI17000.pdf (accessed on November 15, 2013), revised February 2013.

14. Sawada Y et al. Probable toxicity of surface-active agent in commercial herbicide containing glyphosate. Lancet 1(8580), 299, 1988.

15. Lee H et al. Clinical presentations and prognostic factors of a glyphosate–surfactant herbicide intoxication: a review of 131 cases. Acad Emerg Med 7, 234–247, 2000.

16. Temple WA, Smith NA. Glyphosate herbicide poisoning experience in New Zealand. N Z Med J 105, 173–174, 1992.

17. Talbot AR et al. Acute poisoning with a glyphosate-surfactant herbicide ('Roundup'): A review of 93 cases. Hum Exp Toxicol 10, 1–8, 1991.

18. US Environmental Protection Agency 1990. Data evaluation report. Primary eye irritation-rabbits: AGR 33252. Rev. by T.F. McMahon and Y.M. Ioannou. Washington, DC: Nov 9.U.S. EPA. Office of Pesticide Programs. Health Effects Division. 1997. Tox oneliners: Clopyralid (Lontrel). Washington, DC, July 8.

19. Pushnoy LA et al. Herbicide (Roundup) pneumonitis. Chest, 114, 1769–1771, 1998.

20. Goldstein DA et al. Pneumonitis and herbicide exposure. Chest, 116, 1234–1236, 1999.

21. Ho MW, Cummins J. Glyphosate toxic and roundup worse. Sci Soc, 26(12), 2005.

22. Gasnier C et al. Glyphosate-based herbicides are toxic and endocrine disruptors in human cell lines. Toxicology, 262, 184–191, 2009.

23. Benachour N, Séralini G-E. Glyphosate formulations induce apoptosis and necrosis in human umbilical, embryonic, and placental cells. Chem Res Toxicol 22(1), 97–105, 2009.

24. Jamison JP et al. Ventilatory impairment from preharvest retted flax. Brit J Ind Med 43, 809–813, 1986.

25. Boulton DW, Fawcett JP. The pharmacokinetics of levosalbutamol – What are the clinical implications. Clin Pharmacokinet 40, 23–40, 2001.
26. Ungern-Sternberg B et al. Salbutamol premedication in children with a recent respiratory tract infection. Ped Anesthesia 19, 1064–1069, 2009.
27. Patel KR et al. Inhaled ethanolic and aqueous solutions via respimat soft mist inhaler are well-tolerated in asthma patients. Respiration, 73(4), 434–440, 2006.
28. Reznik M et al. Inner-city availability of preservative-containing albuterol. Clin Pediatr, 43, 615–617, 2004.
29. Kim SH, Ahn Y. Anaphylaxis caused by benzalkonium in a Nebulizer solution J Kor Med Sci, 19, 289–290, 2004.
30. Asmus MJ et al. Bronchoconstrictor additives in bronchodilator solutions. J Allerg Clin Immunol, 104(Suppl), S53–S60, 1999.
31. Guide to Coroners and Inquests and Charter for coroner services. 2012. http://www.justice.gov.uk/downloads/burials-and-coroners/guide-charter-coroner.pdf (accessed on November 15, 2013).
32. Boina DJ, Bloomquist JR. Blockage of chloride channels and anion transporters with pesticidal natural products and their synthetic analogs. Phytochem Rev, 10, 217–226, 2011.
33. Thany SH, et al. Identification of cholinergic synaptic transmission in the insect nervous system. Adv Exp Med Biol. 683, 1–10, 2010.
34. Carson R. Silent Spring. Mariner Books, New York, 2002 (First published by Houghton Mifflin, 1962)].
35. Zhang Y et al. Immunotoxicity of pyrethroid metabolites in an in vitro model. Environ Toxicol Chem, 29, 2505–2510, 2010.
36. Zucchini-Pascal N et al. Organochlorine pesticides induce epithelial to mesenchymal transition of human primary cultured hepatocytes. Food Chem Toxicol, 50, 3963–3970, 2012.
37. Zhao X et al. Fipronil is a potent open channel blocker of glutamate-activated chloride channels in cockroach neurons. J Pharmacol Exp Ther 310, 192–201, 2004.
38. Tós-Luty S et al. Dermal and oral toxicity of malathion in rats. Ann Agric Environ Med, 10(1), 101–106, 2003.
39. Lein PJ et al. Genome-wide expression profiling of carbaryl and vinclozolin in human thyroid follicular carcinoma (FTC-238) cells Neurotoxicology, 33, 660–670, 2012.
40. London L et al. Neurobehavioral and neurodevelopmental effects of pesticide exposures. Neurotoxicology, 33(special issue), 887–896, 2012.
41. Blacquiere T et al. Neonicotinoids in bees: a review on concentrations, side-effects and risk assessment Ecotoxicology, 21, 973–992, 2012.
42. Lin PC et al. Acute poisoning with neonicotinoid insecticides: a case report and literature review. Basic Clin Pharmacol Toxicol, 112, 282–286, 2013.
43. Phua DH et al. Neonicotinoid insecticides: an emerging cause of acute pesticide poisoning. Clin Toxicol, 47, 336–341, 2009.
44. Tomizawa M et al. Neonicotinoid insecticide toxicology: mechanisms of selective action. Ann Rev Pharm Toxicol, 45, 247–262, 2005.
45. Ryu HW et al. Amurensin G induces autophagy and attenuates cellular toxicities in a rotenone model of Parkinson's disease. Biochem Biophys Res Comm, 433, 121–126, 2013.

46. Coleman MD et al. A preliminary investigation into the impact of a pesticide combination on human neuronal and glial cell lines in vitro. PLoS One, 7, e42768, 2012.

47. Pesticide Residues in Food. 1997. Report. (FAO Plant Production and Protection Paper – 145) Report of the Joint Meeting of the FAO Panel of Experts on Pesticide Residues in Food and the Environment and the WHO Core Assessment Group on Pesticide Residues Lyons, France 22 September–1 October 1997 World Health Organization Food and Agriculture Organization of the United Nations, Rome, 1998.

48. Kato R et al. Contribution of GABAergic inhibition to the responses of secondary vestibular neurons to head rotation in the rat. Neurosci Res, 46, 499–512, 2003.

49. Valla J et al. Vestibulotrigeminal and vestibulospinal projections in rats: retrograde tracing coupled to glutamic acid decarboxylase immunoreactivity. Neurosci Lett, 340, 225–230, 2003.

50. Magnusson AK et al. 2002. Early compensation of vestibulo-oculomotor symptoms after unilateral vestibular loss in rats is related to GABA (B) receptor function. Neuroscience, 111, 625–630, 2002.

51. Stout DM et al. American Healthy Homes Survey: a national study of residential pesticides measured from floor wipes. Environ Sci Technol 43, 4294–4300, 2009.

52. Lee SJ. Acute illnesses associated with exposure to fipronil—surveillance data from 11 states in the United States, 2001–2007. Clin Toxicol, 48, 737–744, 2010.

53. Jennings KA et al. Human exposure to fipronil from dogs treated with frontline. Vet Hum Toxicol, 44, 301–303, 2002.

54. National Pesticide Information Center. 2009. Fipronil: Technical Fact Sheet. http://npic.orst.edu/factsheets/fiptech.pdf (accessed on November 11, 2013).

55. Mohamed F et al. Acute human self-poisoning with the N-phenylpyrazole insecticide fipronil – a GABA(A)-gated chloride channel blocker. J Toxicol Clin Toxicol, 42, 955–963, 2004.

56. Vidau C et al. Exposure to sublethal doses of fipronil and thiacloprid highly increases mortality of honeybees previously infected by Nosema ceranae. PLoS One, 6(6), e21550, 2011.

57. Lassiter T et al. Is fipronil safer than chlorpyrifos? Comparative developmental neurotoxicity modelled in PC12 cells. Brain Res Bull, 78, 313–322, 2009.

58. Eyer P. Neurophysiological changes by organophosphorus compounds – a review. Hum Exp Toxicol, 14, 857, 1995.

59. Axelrad JC et al. The effects of acute pesticide exposure on neuroblastoma cells chronically exposed to diazinon. Toxicology, 185, 67–72, 2003.

60. Ecobichon DJ, Organophosphorus ester insecticides. In: Ecobichon DJ, Joy RN, editors. Pesticides and Neurological Diseases. CRC Press, Boca Raton, 171–249, 1994.

61. Levin HS, Rodnitzky RL. Behavioral aspects of organophosphate pesticides in man. Clin Toxicol, 9, 391, 1976.

62. Spiegelberg U. Psychopathological and neurological late and later effects of intoxication with organophosphate esters. Proc 14th Congress Occ Health Excerpta Medica, 62, 1963.

63. Cherry N et al. Paroxonase (PON) polymorphisms in farmers attributing ill-health to sheep dip. Lancet, 359, 763–764, 2002.

64. Trainor M et al. Risk assessment for acute toxicity from sheep ectoparasite treatments, including organo phosphates (OPs) used in plunge dipping. Health and Safety Executive Report, HSL/2002/26. Health and Safety Executive, Sheffield, 2002.

65. Garfitt SJ. Oral and dermal exposure to propetamphos: a human volunteer study. Toxicol Lett, 134, 115–118, 2002.

66. Mackness B. Paraoxonase and susceptibility to organophosphorus poisoning in farmers dipping sheep. Pharmacogenetics, 13, 81–88, 2003.

67. Handy RD et al. Chronic diazinon exposure: pathologies of spleen, thymus, blood cells, and lymph nodes are modulated by dietary protein or lipid in the mouse. Toxicology, 172, 13, 2002.

68. Yilmazarlar A, Ozyurt G. Brain involvement in organophosphate poisoning. Environ Res, 74, 104–109, 1997.

69. Rosenstock L et al. The pesticide health effects study group. Lancet, 338, 223–227, 1991.

70. Grob D, Harvey AM. The effects and treatment of nerve gas poisoning. Am J Med, 14, 52–55, 1953.

71. Grob D, Harvey JC. Effects in man of the anticholinesterase compound sarin (isopropyl methylphosphonofluoridate). J Clin Invest, 37, 350–368, 1958.

72. Nakajima T et al. Urinary metabolites of sarin in a patient of the matsumoto sarin incident. Arch Toxicol, 72(9), 601–603, 1998.

73. Korsak RJ, Sato MM. Effects of chronic organophosphate pesticide exposure on the central nervous system. Clin Toxicol, 11, 83–95, 1977

74. Hayes WJ, Jr, Pesticides Studied in Man. Williams & Wilkins, Baltimore, 1982.

75. Poncelet N. An algorithm for the evaluation of peripheral neuropathy. Am Fam Phys 57, 755–764, 1998.

76. O'Neill JJ. Non-cholinesterase effects of anticholinesterases. Fund Appl Toxicol, 1, 1981, 154–160.

77. Clement JG, Copeman HT. Soman and sarin induce a long-lasting naloxone-reversible analgesia in mice. Life Sci, 34, 1415–1422, 1984.

78. Davies DR, Holland P. Effect of oximes and atropine upon the development of delayed neuropathy in chickens following poisoning by DFP and sarin. Biochem Pharmacol, 21, 1972, 3145–3151.

79. Stephens R et al. Organophosphates: the relationship between chronic and acute exposure effects. Neurotoxicol Teratol, 18, 449–453, 1996.

80. Duffy FH, Burchfield JL, Long-term effects of the organophosphate sarin on EEG in monkeys and humans. Neurotoxicology, 1, 667–689, 1980.

81. Stephens R et al. Neuropsychological effects of long-term exposure to organophosphate in sheep dip. The Lancet, 345, 1135–1139, 1995.

82. Jokanovic M et al. Neurotoxic effects in patients poisoned with organophosphorus pesticides. Env Toxicol Pharmacol. 29, 195–201, 2010.

83. Ng TP et al. Neurobehavioral effects of industrial mixed solvent exposure in Chinese printing and paint workers. Neurotoxicol Teratol, 12, 661–664, 1990.

84. Mikkelsen S. Epidemiological update on solvent neurotoxicity. Environ Res, 73, 101–112, 1997.

85. Marrs TC et al. Chemical Warfare Agents, Toxicology and Treatment. John Wiley & Sons, New York, 1996.

86. Klaassen CD, editor. Casarett and Doull's Toxicology: The Basic Science of Poisons, 5th edition. McGraw Hill, New York, 1996.

87. Mendola P et al. Organophosphate pesticide metabolites in urine from preschool children with flu-like illnesses. Epidemiology, 12, 75, 2001.

88. US EPA. 1990. Data Evaluation Report. Primary Eye Irritation-Rabbits: AGR 33252. Rev. by T.F. McMahon and Y.M. Ioannou. Washington, DC, Nov 9.U.S. EPA. Office of Pesticide Programs. Health Effects Division. Tox oneliners: Clopyralid (Lontrel). Washington, DC, July 8, 1997.

89. Kidd H, James DR, editors. The Agrochemicals Handbook, 3rd edition. Royal Society of Chemistry Information Services, Cambridge, 2–13, 1991.

90. Stevens JT, Sumner DD. Herbicides. In: Hayes WJ, Jr, Laws ER, Jr, editors. Handbook of Pesticide Toxicology. Academic Press, New York, 1991, 7–20.

91. Landrigan P et al. 2003. Regional Pesticides Workshop. www.turi.org/community/pdf/GuideChemicalEffects6.pdf (accessed on November 11, 2013).

92. National Library of Medicine Toxnet: Pyrazon: http://toxnet.nlm.nih.gov/cgi-bin/sis/search/a?/dbs+hsdb:@term+@DOCNO+1759 (accessed on November 15, 2013).

93. Williams GM et al. Safety evaluation and risk assessment of the herbicide roundup and its active ingredient, glyphosate, for humans. Regul Toxicol Pharmacol, 31, 117–165, 2000.

94. National Office of Animal Health (NOAH). 2004. Compendium of Data Sheets for Veterinary Products. p 652. NOAH, Enfield, Middlesex.

95. Woods HF (Chairman, Committee on the Toxicity of Chemicals in Food, Consumer Products and the Environment. Organophosphates. Department of Health, London, 1999.

96. Steenland K et al. Chronic neurological sequelae to organophosphate poisoning. Am J Public Health, 84, 731–736, 1994.

97. Johnson AK. Organophosphates and delayed neuropathy – is NTE alive and well? Toxicol Appl Pharmacol, 102, 385–399, 1990.

98. Levin G et al. Anxiety associated with exposure to organophosphate compounds Arch Gen Psychiat, 33, 225–228, 1976.

99. Tabershaw IR, Cooper WC. Sequelae of acute organic phosphate poisoning. J Occup Med, 8, 5–20, 1966.

100. Whorton MD, Obrinsky DL. Persistence of symptoms after mild to moderate acute organophosphate poisoning among 19 farm field workers. J Toxicol Environ Health, 11, 347–354, 1983.

101. Fiedler N et al. Long-term use of organophosphates and neuropsychological performance. Am J Ind Med, 32, 487–496, 1997.

102. Proctor NH et al. Chemical Hazards of the Workplace. J.B. Lippincott Company, Philadelphia, 1988.

103. RTECS, online database U.S. Department of Health and Human Services. 1993. Registry of Toxic Effects of Chemical Substances. National Toxicology Information Program, National Library of Medicine, Bethesda.

104. Surralles J. et al. Induction of micronuclei by 5 pyrethroid insecticides in whole blood and isolated uman lymphocyte cultures. Mutat Res Gen Toxicol. 341, 169–184, 1995.

105. Ray DE. Forshaw PJ. Pyrethroid insecticides: poisoning syndromes, synergies, and therapy. J Toxicol Clin Toxicol, 38(2), 95–101, 2000.

106. van der Merwe D et al. A physiologically based pharmacokinetic model of organophosphate dermal absorption. Toxicol Sci, 89, 188–204, 2006.

107. Nielsen JB, Andersen H. Dermal in vitro penetration of methiocarb, paclobutrazol, and pirimicarb: effect of nonylphenolethoxylate and protective gloves. Environ Health Perspect, 109(2), 129–132, 2001.
108. Sams C et al. Evidence for the activation of organophosphate pesticides by cytochromes P-450 3A4 and 2D6 in human liver microsomes. Toxicol Lett, 116, 217, 2000.
109. Lauriault VV et al. Hepatocyte toxicity induced by various hepatotoxins mediated by cytochrome P-450 IIE1; protection with DDC administration. Chem Biol Int, 81, 271, 1992.
110. British National Formulary. 2013. www.bnf.org/bnf/index.htm (accessed on November 11, 2013).
111. Jamal GA et al. Low level exposures to organophosphorus esters may cause neurotoxicity, Toxicology, 181/182, 23–33, 2002.
112. Terry AV. Functional consequences of repeated organophosphate exposure: potential non-cholinergic mechanisms. Pharmacol Ther, 134, 355–365, 2012.
113. Chen Y. Organophosphate-induced brain damage: mechanisms, neuropsychiatric and neurological consequences, and potential therapeutic strategies Neurotoxicology, 33, 391–400, 2012.

6

Toxicity of imported goods

6.1 Overseas manufactured imported goods: Context

Over the last 25 years, economies in the Far East, such as China, Vietnam, Taiwan and Korea, have grown at a spectacular pace. They have gained huge market shares for their manufactured goods of almost every variety in most developed countries. Whilst this expansion in manufacturing capability has brought employment and burgeoning wealth, the environmental cost in some countries has been extreme and the scale of pollution amongst all sectors of society in parts of China is truly vast. The pollution has even been linked to a decline in the capable Chinese workforce [1] and although dire air quality issues are beginning to be addressed in some cities such as Shanghai [2], exposure to toxins such as lead, for example, is all pervading. Extensive mining and consumption of the metal has led to its release into local ecosystems and foodstuffs, strongly impacting health [1, 3]. The plastics industry in China is particularly large and successful, but over the last decade has been responsible for a disproportional share of product recalls, often due to toxicity linked with its products, such as continued release of solvent vapours, as well as the extensive use of heavy metals in paints and finishes [4, 5]. It is important to realise that the plastics industry worldwide is also associated with an array of potentially toxic agents which impact users, manufacturers and the environment; these include vinyl chloride, styrene as well as polycyclics, phthalates, bisphenol A, the various brominated flame retardants (PBDEs, polybrominated diphenyl ethers) and the so far unknown impact of complex mixtures of the aforementioned agents. These agents are a potent occupational health issue in the developed world [6] and the alarming toxicity of some of the products that emerge from the developing world's plastics industries is an indication that those engaged in manufacturing them are working for organisations and infrastructures which are not aware of even basic standards of worker protection. There is little or no regulation of manufacturing in China and this is coupled with a widespread ignorance of basic occupational toxin knowledge,

Expert Report Writing in Toxicology: Forensic, Scientific and Legal Aspects,
First Edition. Michael D. Coleman.
© 2014 John Wiley & Sons, Ltd. Published 2014 by John Wiley & Sons, Ltd.

which was highlighted earlier in Chapter 3.3, with respect to the use of hexane as a degreaser in computer assembly.

Whilst it is not possible from the developed world to directly influence the plight of workers in unregulated industries in the developing world, it is important to investigate and curtail the sale of goods which are unsafe, in that they might injure or cause toxicity to consumers in the developed world. If sales of such goods are impacted by these measures, then it is to be hoped that this will employ economic forces to eventually feedback onto developing world manufacturing practices to make them less dangerous to their workforces and more environmentally sustainable in the future.

6.2   Reports for trading standards

Whilst vast amounts of imported goods are sold in the United Kingdom every year, relatively few are evaluated to the degree that their potential toxicity might be revealed. Often, concerns are raised by complaints from the public, which are investigated by Local Council Trading Standards Officers. Once the agent has been examined, to justify a request to the imported to curtail importation of an article, a short expert report may be required to highlight the hazards present in the product and its implications for its distribution to the public. The Trading Standards Officers may go as far as to institute court proceedings against suppliers and distributors of particularly unsafe or toxic imported articles. Due to a combination of very low overseas manufacturing and shipping costs, distributing imported goods in the United Kingdom can be extremely profitable, so importers may actively resist attempts to withdraw such goods from high street and internet retail outlets. Hence, an expert report can be very valuable in persuading a court that the agents do pose sufficient risk to the public for them to be withdrawn from sale.

The following short reports provide some idea of the range of different articles available which have contravened regulations on safety and the nature of their particular hazards.

6.3   Plastic tank: Naphthalene

Local Trading Standards consulted me over a plastic tank imported from China, which was approximately $14 \times 8 \times 8$ in. and was a substantial toy. The purchaser had alerted Trading Standards, due to the powerful chemical smell emanating from the plastic of the toy. Upon analysis, this was found mostly to be naphthalene and a senior Trading Standards Officer brought the tank to my office for inspection. Fortunately, no students visited my office at that time, as they would have been greeted with the sight of two grown men apparently playing with a particularly smelly, large plastic tank. Over the years, there have been many complaints world-wide over the strong polycyclic aromatic hydrocarbon vapours emanating from a variety of Chinese-sourced containers, toys and even clothing. Naphthalene is flammable and this is its primary hazard in this context. The dose that might be ingested by a child using the toy in a confined space on a regular basis is difficult to quantify. However, there is a long list of hazards associated with this solvent, as it is toxic to the skin, causing quite severe irritation in some individuals. In addition, it is easily absorbed through inhalation and is an ocular toxin [7]. In addition to its carcino-genicity in experimental animals, there would have been a considerable risk of local irritation to a child's skin and eyes if they played with the tank regularly. The article was subsequently withdrawn from sale.

6.4   Soft toys: Phthalates

Trading Standards may carry out checks on a variety of soft toys to ensure that they comply with current importation regulations. During a routine check of several swimming aids, plastic animals and dinosaurs, as well as other articles, they were found to contain phthalates. These agents were banned from children's toys in January 2007 in the United Kingdom, but these articles were confiscated more than 14 months after the ban had come into force. I was asked to supply some background information to aid the composition of the press release associated with Trading Standard's actions in withdrawing the toys. Phthalates are a significant worldwide problem from several perspectives. It was discovered that they make plastics more pliable and easy to mould, work and enhance functionality. With the expansion of the plastics industry, their manufacture has burgeoned to around a quarter of a million tonnes worldwide every year. Importantly from a toxicological perspective, they are not covalently bound to the plastic matrix, which means that they escape during use and enter the user's body or leach out of landfills into groundwater after they are discarded. Finally, much evidence has accumulated that they are toxic endocrine disruptors, which cause profound derangement of reproductive cycles and fertility in humans and other species and they have other disruptive effects, such as oxidative stressor actions [8]. Not surprisingly, toy manufacturers did not welcome the banning of phthalates in children's toys [9, 10], particularly di-(2-ethyl hexyl) phthalate (DEHP), diethyl phthalate (DEP), dibutyl phthalate (DBP) and benzyl butyl phthalate (BBP). Indeed, Chinese manufacturers, which make around 85% of the world's toys, still run production lines without the agents incorporated, for export to the European Union and United States, whilst other lines continue to make products containing these toxins aimed at countries which still allow these chemicals. As more evidence of the toxicity of phthalates emerges and more countries ban them, products containing phthalates will become exceedingly cheap and importers may well be misled on their provenance, so the danger of toys entering the

United Kingdom and European Union which contain these toxins remains present for the foreseeable future.

6.5   Wooden toy story one: Barium and lead

I was contacted again by the same Trading Standards Office over a wooden counting frame, which was rather like an abacus. The toy, which was of Chinese origin, was examined for metal content of the paint and found to exceed the maximum limits by a high margin. Interestingly, prior to their approach to myself, Trading Standards had tried to have this toy withdrawn by the importer, who resisted this move, by commissioning a report from a medical doctor (Dr XY) which stated that the toys posed no threat to children. The basis of his argument was that so-called 'barium meals' used in radiocontrast examinations of gastrointestinal tract problems were perfectly safe, so barium in paint must also be safe. However, this observation was erroneous and needed to be refuted before Trading Standards could bring a case against the importer. Dr XY's background was in medicine and he made the assumption that his medical experience with barium also applied to other forms of the metal. In report writing it is clearly essential to make no unwarranted assumptions and to check all information as thoroughly as possible. Although mistakes will always be made, better that they are trivial rather than substantial.

Returning to the case, it is not enough just to state that the toy in question might be a problem in principle. Specifically and from a practical standpoint, some calculated projection is necessary to estimate what possible amounts of the metal might be ingested by a child and what would be the range of medical impact that might be experienced. Whilst such calculations are estimates and might be reasonably open to challenge in court or by another expert, it does provide a plausible basis upon which to argue that the toy represents a clear potential danger to some children and the impact on the community might be proportional to the toy's popularity.

> The report started with the usual qualifications and background suitability to build credibility.
>
> On 22 May 2002 Mr Z, an Assistant Trading Standards Officer of XXXX MBC Trading Standards Division drew my attention to a Wooden Counting Frame identified with sample reference number 513316 where the paints used to coat this toy had been demonstrated by Birmingham City Laboratories to have exceeded the recognised limits of permitted migration for barium by more than sevenfold and the limits for lead by nearly twofold. No other heavy metals were detected. I was asked to comment on the potential toxicity of the major contaminant, barium, and to make some assessment of any risk this toy might pose to a child.

Nature of barium

1. Barium is a divalent alkaline-earth metal of such high reactivity that it can spontaneously ignite when exposed to moist air. Consequently, it is only found in nature
   as stable salts. Barium ore is known as barite, which is barium sulphate; the carbonate is used in glass-making, the chlorate and nitrate are constituents of some
   fireworks. Although there are a variety of uses of barium salts, all are toxic and
   their toxicity is directly related to their solubility in water.

Barium absorption

1. The amount of barium that will enter a child's body, in the case of this toy, depends
   on a number of factors. The solubility of barium is greatest when it is present as a
   chloride, much less when it is sulphate and practically zero as a carbonate. Large
   doses of barium sulphate are administered routinely orally as a contrast agent in the
   visualisation of the gastrointestinal tract. As barium sulphate is virtually insoluble,
   the metal itself does not detectably enter the blood and thus barium enemas/barium
   'meals', etc. are not associated with any danger of barium metal toxicity, except
   when they are inadvertently inhaled [11].

2. It is not widely known, however, that soluble forms of the metal such as the chloride enter the blood rapidly when taken by mouth. Barium absorbed into the bloodstream leaves within a day or so, entering the muscles, lungs and bone. It can be
   found in the muscles around two days after absorption and eventually it is slowly
   excreted.

3. As barium is a divalent metal it is treated in a similar fashion to calcium in the body
   and certainly in children, with their demand for calcium for bone and dental growth,
   their barium uptake and subsequent tissue availability, its soluble form would be
   greater than that of adults. The deposition of barium into bone is similar to calcium
   but occurs at a faster rate [12].

Barium effects

1. The half-life of barium in bone is estimated to be about 50 days [13]. The effects
   of barium toxicity are as follows: (i) Cardiovascular system: sub-chronic to chronic
   symptoms include increased blood pressure, disturbance of potassium blood concentrations and increased incidence of cardiovascular disease in humans. An acute
   overdose can result in cardiac irregularities. Convulsions and death from cardiac
   and respiratory failure can occur. (ii) Nervous system: acute to sub-chronic symptoms include weakness, tremors, anxiety and breathing problems. An acute overdose can result in convulsions and death from cardiac and respiratory failure. (iii)
   Gastrointestinal system: acute to sub-chronic symptoms include excess salivation,
   vomiting, and diarrhoea in humans.

2. The possible effects of barium in children in this context are as follows: of the few
   studies that have been carried out in barium's effects in man, Wones et al. [14]

found that a level of 10 mg/L (0.21 mg/kg/day) dose over 10 weeks could be tolerated, yielding no observable effects in male adults. For a 20 kg child, this translates to 4.2 mg of soluble barium per day. This assumes that children show a similar sensitivity to barium compared with adults. It is often the case that children are much more sensitive to metal toxicity compared with adults. Lead is a prime example of this, where convulsions can be caused in children at doses which are easily tolerated by adults.

Potential transfer of barium

1. Since the toy in question can yield 7 mg of soluble barium per gramme of paint according to the Birmingham City Laboratory Analysis, ingestion of 1 gramme of the paint by a 20 kg child could result in the no-effect level of barium exposure being exceeded by 175%. This value would be even higher in a 10–15 kg child. Although this would be a short-term toxicity, conservatively, it could lead to diarrhoea and general gastrointestinal upset and at worst, if the child had an underlying heart condition, it is possible that exposure to this level of barium could exacerbate this condition. The child could ingest the paint by damaging the toy and ingesting the beads whole, so the paint is leeched off the beads in the stomach; alternatively, the child may chew the beads to scrape off the paint.

2. My comments on Dr XY's report are as follows: Although Dr XY has not seen any cases of barium poisoning in children, it does occur; for example, when barium in rat poison has been inadvertently used in cooking [15]. It is apparent from reading his report that Dr XY is unaware that barium can exist in soluble forms and that its toxicity is directly related to its water solubility. I agree that the level of lead in the counting frame would probably not be significant in this case, but Dr XY was also unaware that the major source of lead for children, even today, is their diet. This is particularly problematic in poor, disadvantaged areas, where lead piping is still used and reliance on canned food is much higher than in more prosperous locations.

3. Metal toxicity in general is more acute in children who are poorly nourished, as their digestive systems upregulate absorption of divalent metals, such as lead and barium, in a bid to boost calcium levels. Overall, the amount of toxin yielded from a toy has to be seen in the context of the children's current exposure to metals according to their location and socio-economic background. Dr XY does not believe that a child could ingest enough of the paint to show any ill-effects. However, it is not beyond the realms of possibility that the toy could be broken (it is made of wood) and the beads swallowed. In addition, it is common knowledge that children do bite and chew various articles and it is also possible that they could chew the paint off this toy.

4. In my opinion, the levels of barium found in the paint on this toy are entirely unacceptable and I would not allow my own child to use it. There is sufficient bioavailable barium in the toy to cause toxicity to a child that ingested the paint, and therefore the toy does pose a risk to health which should not be tolerated in a toy aimed and marketed at young children.

I understand that my duty is to assist on matters within my expertise, namely bio-chemical toxicology. This duty overrides any obligations to the person from whom instructions or payment have been received. In writing this report I have complied with this duty and I believe the facts I have stated herein are true and the opinions I have expressed are correct.

M.D. Coleman

6.5.1   Case comment

The Distributors challenged this report in a letter, where they took issue with my credibility regarding my opinion and that of a paediatrician, that the toys would be attractive to children. They also worded their letter in such a way to suggest that the fault lay with the child and their parents for allowing them to lick or suck the toys, which would be perfectly safe in their view, provided they were not chewed. On this logic, it would be permissible to manufacture children's toys from asbestos, provid-ing the children and their parents signed a written undertaking not to bore into, grind or otherwise deploy abrasives of any description upon the said (non-flammable, of course) toy. Their letter carried on to suggest that if indeed children were likely to ingest the metal contaminants, then this would not pose a significant problem. There were no actual arguments supplied to support this contention. They also rather blatantly misrepresented my calculation arguments to suggest that I had actu-ally approved of the level of soluble barium in the toys.

None of this changed the fact that the level of soluble barium in the toys was seven times the legal maximum and was in breach of Trading Standards regulations. The agent is toxic and was potentially systemically bioavailable. The earlier brief report was used in Trading Standards' prosecution of the Distributors who decided to plead guilty in the local magistrate's court. They were fined £2000 for marketing toys with excessive metal contents, costs were awarded against them and, interest-ingly, the Distributors were also fined for fraudulently placing a 'CE' mark to the toy, which suggested that the toy had European Community approval.

6.6   Wooden toy story two: Chromium and lead

Trading Standards invited me to write another report concerning a toy which was similar to the earlier case, in that the items were made of wood and contained approximately sixfold the recommended lead and chromium contents in their paint. Despite the submission of my report and Trading Standards efforts, the Distributor resisted all attempts to have the toys withdrawn. Trading Standards took them to their local Magistrates Court and the Distributor fought the case vigorously, hence barristers were employed on both sides. It soon became apparent that the reason the Distributors thought it worth fighting the case was that their counsel used arguments deployed in the earlier case with the barium-contaminated toys. They stated that the items were not actually legally classifiable as toys, rather, they were decorations and thus exempt from the usual regulations regarding paint metal content. In addition, their counsel also contended that the levels of the paints did not pose a realistic toxic risk in the context of everyday life. To counter these two arguments, Trading Standards called a paediatrician to examine the decorations and write a short report on the attractiveness of the items to children as well as their toxicity. I was to be called to comment on the estimation of toxic risk. The paediatrician was called to give evidence and was cross-examined by the Distributor's barrister. He maintained a strong line that the items were attractive to children in his professional opinion and would be likely to be played with, chewed and otherwise damaged in such a way that the metals could be ingested by a child.

I was called to give evidence and the line the barrister took was essentially that life was a toxic risk *per se* and that the metals in the paint were not really a significant addition to the general toxic burden of life. Although I had been introduced to the court as Dr Coleman, he continually referred to me as Mr Coleman, despite repeated corrections. This may have been merely an oversight or a concerted attempt to disrupt my composure. Given the elaborate and precise courtesies normally observed between barristers, magistrates and judges during court business, it was more likely to be the latter scenario. During my 45 minutes or so in the witness box, I argued that the metal levels in the paint were some way outside what would be interpreted as a 'normal toxic burden' and such specific toxicity was not justified in my opinion. I also perhaps emphasised repeatedly the known cancer risks associated with chromium and mentioned that there was really no safe exposure to a potential carcinogen, especially in children, who are developing and are vulnerable to such toxicity. Since the magistrates looked around the age where they may have had young grandchildren, it is likely that this point would not have gone unnoticed.

The barrister did attempt to manipulate what I had said in my report to a minor degree, but he was essentially hamstrung as it did not appear that the Distributor had commissioned its own expert opinion on the toxicity of the paints. Indeed, they had no causation expertise other than their legal team's interpretations. The Trading Standards barrister was extremely effective in arguing, with no small measure of panache, that the decorations were a toxic risk to children and that they should be withdrawn. The Magistrates agreed with him and awarded costs to Trading Standards. From the look on his face, it was clear that the opposing barrister was far from happy with the result, as he had been dispatched, as World War II Luftwaffe fighter pilots used to say, *mit eleganz*. The Distributor was fined several thousand pounds and was forced to pay legal costs. More to the point, it was denied the future profits from what had been a lucrative, if somewhat toxic line of merchandise.

6.7 Adhesives: Chloroform

In the popular imagination, chloroform is most closely associated with grainy monochrome film noir, when the hapless wasp-waisted heroine is chloroformed by some wicked kidnapper sporting a black fedora and a double-breasted pin-striped suit with implausibly wide lapels. Given its somewhat dubious reputation, the use of chloroform in a domestic adhesive seems bizarre; however, it is perceived by manufacturers in product design that they must utilise chemicals which are reasonably cheap but that they also conform to basic standards of safety. One of the primary issues with solvents in any application is their combination of volatility and flammability, and chloroform is not perceived as flammable. However, this means that whilst it does not burn with the heat of, say methyl isobutyl ketone, which is used in Police CS sprays, it nevertheless does decompose into toxic products during pyrolysis as will be seen later and it is entirely unacceptable as the base for any adhesive to be used in any context, domestic or industrial. I was asked to provide a report on several adhesives which contained this solvent by a local Trading Standards Office.

The Toxicity of Chloroform in Various Supplied Superglues

A report to XXXX Trading Standards written by: Professor Michael Coleman, B.Sc., Ph.D., D.Sc., F.H.E.A.

Properties of chloroform

1. Chloroform is found as a very volatile non-flammable liquid at room temperature. It has a characteristic sweet odour and a high vapour pressure, which means that its odour quickly distributes in a room when a container of the substance is left open. It will boil at only 61–62 °C and it is quite reactive chemically. If it is subject to heat, such as from an open flame, it decomposes to form the toxic gas phosgene, which was used as an effective battlefield chemical weapon in the Great War. This gas causes extreme irritation to the lungs, which results in sufficiently high mucous production to cause asphyxiation *in extremis*. When heated, chloroform can also cause the release of chlorine gas, which is also intensely irritating to the respiratory system [16, 17].

Uses

1. Chloroform was mainly used to make chlorofluorocarbons, which were responsible for ozone depletion and their use has predictably declined in the refrigeration industry. The lack of flammability of chloroform led to its use in fire extinguishers, which has also been discontinued. The agent remains as a solvent as part of the chemical industry, as well as in analytical and synthetic chemistry laboratories. It is also part of the production of pesticides, dyes and cosmetics. Its toxicity has been recognised for over 30 years and alternative solvents have been utilised in many industries to gradually replace this agent and reduce the risks of human toxicity.

'Normal' human exposure

1. Currently, the main exposure to chloroform is in drinking water, as it is formed from the chlorination process. Exposure was measured in the 1970s to be in the range of 0.02–0.07 ppm [18] and there is also evidence that it is detectable in the atmosphere at much lower levels (0.00004 ppm). This latter exposure is related to industrial production and will vary according to the site of measurement. Chloroform exposure in food is due to the use of tap water in processing. The concentrations of chloroform which might normally be expected for 'normal' human exposure are thus likely around the 0.03–0.05 ppm range, which is less than half what is generally regarded as the lowest chloroform concentration which is non-hazardous (0.5 mg/m^3; or 0.1 ppm [18]).

2. The greater the level this concentration of chloroform exposure is exceeded, the more likely there will be adverse health consequences. UK legal limits for eight hour workplace exposure of chloroform are somewhat higher than the US limits (2 ppm or 9.9 mg mg/m^3 [19]). Given that the US limits have been set with reference to extensive animal studies, these are likely to be more realistic in their estimation of potential chloroform toxicity in man.

Routes of entry

1. Chloroform is very lipophilic (soluble in oils) so it penetrates skin and more than 70% is absorbed from inhalation. It is rapidly absorbed when ingested orally and is metabolised to a series of toxic species such as phosgene and other carbonyl derivatives [20] which may cause liver necrosis after both chronic and acute exposure.

Acute human toxicity

1. Chloroform is known popularly as being capable of anaesthetisation and it can induce unconsciousness at levels as low as 1500 ppm. Death may occur at levels exceeding 30–40,000 ppm due to central nervous system (CNS) depression. At levels below 1500 ppm the chemical may cause CNS effects such as dizziness, tiredness and ataxia (staggering gait). Fatalities have resulted from the ingestion of as little as 10 mL of chloroform, the cause of death being cardiac arrest [21]. Other acute effects include increase heart and respiratory rates, nausea, vomiting and confusion.

Abuse

2. Owing to its CNS effects, chloroform has been known for more than a century [22] to have the potential for abuse, which has been widely recognised with other products containing volatile organic solvents. Its characteristic effects include euphoria, hallucinations and usually severe vomiting following cessation of use.

Chronic human toxicity

1. Chronically, chloroform is known to cause a series of CNS-related effects which are common to many organic solvents, ranging from depression, irritability, as well as hepatitis and jaundice in abusers of the chemical [23]. There is evidence in animal studies that chloroform is carcinogenic [24], particularly to the kidney and liver. It is now classed as a Group B2 (probable human carcinogen) agent by the US Environmental Protection Agency [23].

Recent research – chloroform cardiotoxicity

1. Although the majority of the health issues related to chloroform were extensively studied up to the end of the 1970s and 1980s, recent work has revealed that the agent is also capable of causing the same lethal cardiotoxicity that led to the restriction of the over the counter (OTC) popular antihistamine Triludan™ (terfenadine) to prescription only medicine (POM) status. How this occurs is as follows. Briefly, the activity of the human heart during normal function is recordable as the 'PQRST' wave process on an electrocardiogram. This describes the process of the heart muscle contracting and recovering before the next contraction.

2. At least 30 drugs, as well as chloroform, inhibit a particular ion channel in the heart known as hERG, which, if disrupted, causes a prolonged interval between the Q and the T points of the electrocardiogram. This means that the heart cannot recover sufficiently before the next contraction and the ventricles go 'out of synch' and the heart becomes more and more disorganised in its pumping sequence (ventricular arrhythmia) and then stops. This can occur within a few minutes of exposure to the chemical which affects the hERG channel. Chloroform can make the effect of any particular chemical or drug that causes this process worse through an additive effect, so exposure to the solvent has the potential in some individuals to cause or accelerate heart failure.

Those at greatest risk from long QT syndrome include women of reproductive age and those taking drugs which cause the effect, such as Triludan™ and amiodarone, an antiarrhythmic agent [25, 26].

Supplied superglues for assessment

The proprietary superglues that have been presented to me for examination by Mr K of XXXX Trading Standards contain chloroform by weight ranging from 10–16%, as analysed by a local Public Analyst.

Glue	Wt of glue (g)	chloroform (mg)
Lifetime classics superglue:	3	492
(Sample No. 604791)		

Better life superglue	3	483
(Sample No. 604786)		
Rapide superglue	25	2575
(Sample No. 604788)		

Projected estimates of exposure: These are made assuming the glues were used in their entirety over a period of 30 minutes in a living/bedroom room of average volume ($\sim 50\,m^3$) which was not ventilated. Ambient temperature is assumed to be $25\,°C$, humidity, approximately 70%.

Lifetime Classics Superglue (604791)

About 492 mg of chloroform distributed in $50\,m^3$ may lead to $9.84\,mg/m^3$. This translates to 19.7 times the safe recommended exposure to chloroform ($0.5\,mg/m^3$) as detailed by the US EPA. This translates as only 1% outside UK workplace limits.

Better Life Superglue (604786)

About 483 mg of chloroform distributed in $50\,m^3$ may lead to $9.66\,mg/m^3$. This translates to 19.3 times the safe recommended exposure to chloroform ($0.5\,mg/m^3$) as detailed by the US EPA. This translates as only 3% outside of UK workplace limits.

Rapide Superglue (604788)

About 2575 mg of chloroform distributed in $50\,m^3$ may lead to $51.5\,mg/m^3$. This translates to 103.0 times the safe recommended exposure to chloroform ($0.5\,mg/m^3$) as detailed by the US EPA. This translates as exceeding UK workplace limits by a factor of 5.2.

Summary

Although complete use of the glues in 30 minutes is a 'worst case scenario' this might be exacerbated by other factors such as a significantly higher temperature maintained in the room, or a more extreme problem such as deliberate ingestion of the product. All three glues would yield total chloroform exposures which are several times the US recognised safe level. In the case of the Better Life Superglue, this is two orders of magnitude or more than 100 times the US safe level and more than five times the UK workplace limit over eight hours.

Taken together, chloroform as detected in the levels present in the Public Analyst's report poses several dangers:

- Release of toxic gases (phosgene/chlorine) if subject to open flame;

- Potential for chronic damage to the liver and kidney;

- Danger of induction of heart failure in certain individuals who may be predisposed to long QT syndrome by either their use of prescription drugs, their sex or their genetic makeup.

Opinion

In my opinion, I do not consider chloroform a safe enough agent to be included in a household product such as superglue and I also believe that the glues pose a threat to health which is sufficiently high that they should be withdrawn from sale on a permanent basis.

M.D. Coleman

6.7.1   Case comment

The glues were withdrawn from sale, but it is likely that they are still being sold in many other countries which do not have rigorous standards related to consumer health and welfare. In general, there are many forces which have propelled the substitution of different solvents in industrial processes for alternative agents. The dangers posed by the chlorofluorocarbon solvents to the ozone layer, as well as their toxicity, led to the use of other agents to achieve the necessary standards of degreasing for the successful completion of manufacturing processes. However, as discussed in Chapter 3 (section 3), the main features of solvents which make them desirable in manufacturing and adhesive usage, volatility and lipophilicity, virtually guarantee penetration into the lung and entrance into the CNS. As outlined in Chapter 2 (section 15), alternatives were sought in the late 1990s to replace several chlorinated solvents as degreasers. Many non-chlorinated solvent systems have been evaluated, such as Dowclene 1601 which is alcohol based [27]. One such replacement solvent was *n*-propyl bromide (1-bromopropane) which has been approved by US Aircraft manufacturer Boeing as a base for high specification vapour degreasing processes (Boeing Specification BAC5408). The agent has also gained acceptance as an adhesive base in many applications. However, there is increasing evidence that *n*-propyl bromide does have issues related to chronic human toxicity such as possible DNA damage, as well as CNS and other effects [28–30]. It has certainly been shown to be acutely neurotoxic on excessive exposure in the absence of protective measures [31]. Therefore, if such an agent is selected for its lack of carcinogenicity or its possible 'green' environmentally friendly associations, it is of course vital that workers are not exposed to excessive quantities of this agent and the full implications of this solvent's impact on health should be elucidated. Ironically, with the case of several chlorinated solvents, it has been found over the years that many of the alternatives are not only inadequate for the task, but are just as toxic or in some cases worse. One approach is for industrial concerns to circumvent the problem through investing in sealed vacuum-controlled high-technology facilities to eliminate 'fugitive' emissions of these solvents, as well as worker contact, so effectively protecting the workforce and the environment simultaneously. This has allowed concerns such as BAE Systems to continue to use chlorinated solvents sufficiently efficiently that they cause less environmental impact than aqueous systems [27].

6.8 Summary

There are several common features in the cases discussed in this chapter. Clearly, a considerable amount of material imported from non-European Union countries into the United Kingdom and Europe is potentially hazardous to customers. Unfortunately, the process whereby Trading Standards monitors these products is largely dependent on the same customers reporting problems with the articles they have bought. It is a herculean task to investigate all the millions of items imported annually and Trading Standards have limited resources, so it is likely that much toxic material will continue to enter the country. It is also apparent that many importers are prepared to defend their right to market products of disputed safety in court if necessary, at considerable cost to themselves and the taxpayer, if they are successful. This is of course because the merchandising of such articles is a very lucrative process, given that shipping and manufacturing costs are so low, in comparison with goods manufactured in the European Union, which are of course subject to stringent regulation. Trading Standards personnel continue to work extremely hard to prevent toxic or dangerous articles reaching the UK consumer, and it is vital that experts are prepared to support them in this onerous but necessary task. From the perspective of worker's rights in developing countries, it could be surmised that products which are not safe to sell in the United Kingdom and Europe are certainly not safe to manufacture, wherever in the world this occurs.

References

1. Yang J. et al. Labour supply and pollution in China. App Econ Lett. 20, 949–952, 2013.
2. Zhao Q. Analysis of air quality variability in Shanghai using AOD and API data in the recent decade Front. Earth Sci. 7, 159–168, 2013.
3. Luo W et al. Effects of chronic lead exposure on functions of nervous system in Chinese children and developmental rats. Neurotoxicology 33, 862–871, 2012.
4. CPSC. Children's Apparel Network Recalls Fleece Hoodie and T-Shirt Sets Due to Violation of Lead Paint Standard; Sold Exclusively at Target, October 17, 2012. http://www.cpsc.gov/cpscpub/prerel/prhtml13/13008.html (accessed on 11 November 2013).
5. CPSC. Captain Cutlass Pirate Toy Guns Recalled by Dillon Importing Due to Violation of Lead Paint Standard, 2012. http://www.cpsc.gov/cpscpub/prerel/prhtml12/12285.html (accessed on 11 November 2013).

6. De Matteo R et al., Chemical exposures of women workers in the plastics industry with particular reference to breast cancer and reproductive hazards. New Solut. 22, 427–448, 2012.

7. Wakefield JC. Naphthalene. CHAPD HQ, UK Health Protection Agency, 2007.

8. Mankidya R et al. Biological impact of phthalates. Toxicol Lett. 217 50–58, 2013.

9. Consumer Product Safety Improvement Act of 2008; Sec. 108. Prohibition on sale of certain products containing specified phthalates. http://www.cpsc.gov// PageFiles/129663/cpsia.pdf (accessed on 11 November 2013).

10. European Union 2005/84/EC of 14 December 2005. http://eur-lex.europa.eu/ LexUriServ/LexUriServ.do?uri=OJ:L:2005:344:0040:0043:en:PDF (accessed on 11 November 2013).

11. McCauley PT, Washington IS. Barium bioavailability as the chloride, sulphate or carbonate salt in the rat. Drug Chem Toxicol. 6(2), 209–217, 1983.

12. Beliles RP. The metals. In: Clayton GD, Clayton FE, editors. Patty's Industrial Hygiene and Toxicology, 4th edition. John Wiley & Sons, New York, 1925–1929, 1994.

13. Machata G. Barium. In: Seiler HG, Sigel H, editors. Handbook on Toxicity of Inorganic Compounds. Marcel Dekker, Inc., New York, 97–101, 1988.

14. Wones RG, Stadler BL, Frohman LA. Lack of effect of drinking water barium on cardiovascular risk factor. Environ Health Perspect. 85, 1–13, 1990.

15. Johnson CH, Van Tassell VJ. Acute barium poisoning with respiratory failure and rhabdomyolysis. Ann Emer Med. 20, 1138–1142, 1991.

16. National Institute for Occupational Safety & Health (NIOSH). Revised Recommended Chloroform Standard. US Department of Health Education and Welfare. US Government Printing Office, Washington, DC, 1979a.

17. NIOSH. Occupational Exposure to Chloroform. Criteria for a Recommended Standard. HEW Publication No. (NIOSH) 75–114. US Department of Health, Education and Welfare. US Government Printing Office, Washington, DC, 1979b.

18. Agency for Toxic Substances and Disease Registry (ATSDR). Toxicological Profile for Chloroform. U.S. Department of Health and Human Services, Public Health Service, Atlanta, 1997.

19. Health and Safety Executive, EH40/2005 Workplace exposure limits Table 1: List of approved workplace exposure limits (as consolidated with amendments). http:// www.hse.gov.uk/coshh/table1.pdf (2007) (accessed on 11 November 2013).

20. Winslow SG, Gerstner HB. Toxicity of chloroform. Drug Chem Toxicol. 1, 259, 1978.

21. U.S. Department of Health and Human Services. 1993. Hazardous Substances Data Bank (HSDB, online database). National Toxicology Information Program, National Library of Medicine, Bethesda.

22. Anonymous: The chloroform habit as described by one of its victims. Detroit Lancet. 8(1884–1885), 251–254. http://www.druglibrary.org/schaffer/history/ e1880/chloroformhabit.htm (accessed on 11 November 2013).

23. US Environmental Protection Agency. http://www.epa.gov/ttn/atw/hlthef/chlorofo. html#ref2,2008 (accessed on 11 November 2013).

24. Davidson IWF et al. Carcinogenicity of chloroform in the rat. Drug Chem. Toxicol. 5, 259, 1978.

25. Lyons MA et al. Computational toxicology of chloroform: reverse dosimetry using Bayesian inference, Markov chain Monte Carlo simulation, and human biomonitoring data. Env Health Persp 116(8), 1040–1046, 2008.

26. Coleman MD. Human Drug Metabolism: An Introduction, 2nd edition pp360, Wiley International, Chichester, UK, 2010.
27. Allcock A. 'Trike' on trial'. *Machinery*, May 2012. www.machinery.co.uk/machinery-features/trichloroethylene-reach-candidate-list-authorisation-safechem-kumi-pero/41878/ (accessed on 11 November 2013).
28. Toraason M et al. DNA damage in leukocytes of workers occupationally exposed to 1-bromopropane. Mutat Res. 603, 1–14, 2006.
29. Frasch HF et al. In vitro human epidermal penetration of 1-bromopropane. J Tox Env Health, Part A, 74, 1249–1260, 2011.
30. Ichihara G et al. A survey on exposure level, health status, and biomarkers in workers exposed to 1-bromopropane. Am J Indust Med. 45, 63–75, 2004.
31. Samukawa M. A case of severe neurotoxicity associated with exposure to 1-bromopropane, an alternative to ozone-depleting or global-warming solvents. Arch Int Med. 172, 1257–1260, 2012.

Epilogue: Occupational health – future perspectives

E.1 The developed world

All of the case studies described in this book were written between 1998 and 2009 and were concerned with exposure to toxins in the United Kingdom as far back as more than half a century in some individuals. Whilst it is clear that the risks of health damage related to occupation remain real even in the developed world, it is hoped that this book also describes how these victims of their occupation have tried to seek redress in a slow and adversarial but ultimately not entirely unreasonable system. Prospective claimants have access to many independent regional bodies which can provide occupational health advice, as described in Chapter 2. There is also a clear legal framework upon which to call to account those who have ignored worker's health, by either negligence or deliberate action. The legal process also discourages those who wish to profit unfairly from Occupational Health issues, by exaggerating or even fabricating their symptoms. It is not perfect, but over the last two centuries, this system has evolved in the United Kingdom whereby those who have suffered health damage through their work can make claims, and a vast international medical research literature is available to help experts establish causation.

Considering future occupational injury trends in the United Kingdom, most would agree that eventually, through the passage of time the numbers of victims of the hazardous industries of the 1940s–1980s will dwindle, and hopefully their claims are processed and settlements made. The industries themselves went into steep decline from the 1970s onwards due to a variety of external factors, such as foreign competition, as well as internal factors, such as those discussed in Chapter 4 concerning the car industry. The response in the United Kingdom in the early 1980s to this decline of heavy industry and manufacturing was to effectively kick away whatever financial crutches were supporting them (at immense social cost) and to attempt to re-direct the economy away from the manufacturing sector towards services and financial systems. This ruthlessly Darwinian and extremely

Expert Report Writing in Toxicology: Forensic, Scientific and Legal Aspects,
First Edition. Michael D. Coleman.
© 2014 John Wiley & Sons, Ltd. Published 2014 by John Wiley & Sons, Ltd.

controversial process had the effect of paring the United Kingdom's manufacturing base down to probably its lowest post-industrial revolution level. The industries that did survive gradually transformed their working environments, to the point where hazard levels are perhaps lower today than they have ever been. This has come about through a combination of factors, such as the emergence of an effective Health and Safety culture, evolution and investment in automation and production development, alongside the use of more efficient manufacturing processes and safer handling of raw materials. Logically, such developments should bring us towards a very significant reduction in cases of occupationally induced health damage in the United Kingdom, and perhaps it might even be hoped that in the intermediate and long-term future, such damage could even be consigned to history.

Such a utopian view would naturally be naïve, partly because of world events over the past decade. The severe economic difficulties of the 2008/2009 'credit crunch' in Western countries has led to a significant contraction in funding for public sector employment, which in the United Kingdom had absorbed many of the workforces made redundant from the moribund manufacturing and heavy industries of the 1980s. Since 2009, in the United Kingdom, Government has sought to foster the process where the Private Sector might provide more employment to offset the reduction in public sector capacity. One of the ways this can be achieved is in promoting manufacturing, which hopefully should not only provide secure, sustainable and well-paid jobs but will generate real wealth which can be taxed to improve the United Kingdom's finances. It could be said in support of this strategy that the great industries of the past such as the car industry started as small concerns, such as making bicycles. Therefore, it should be theoretically possible to seed today more oak trees of the future, so to speak. If successful, such a notion might conceivably lead to a sustained revival of high-quality manufacturing in the country that gave birth to the Industrial Revolution. New industrial processes are appearing which exploit raw materials in ways that are competitive and profitable, but as mentioned in Chapter 1, Health and Safety concerns and expert advice must be sought to ensure that worker's health is safeguarded throughout the industrial process design. Of course, it is not a perfect world, and unforeseen hazards will still arise due to new chemical entities, processes or techniques. However, in the United Kingdom and in the developed world, such cases will be investigated, justice will usually be done regarding culpability and lessons for future exposure will be learned.

E.2   The developing world

Such optimism is not applicable concerning many developing world exporting economies. As mentioned at the beginning of Chapter 6, the sheer pace of industrialisation in many of these countries is remarkable and is perhaps reminiscent of the last 20 years of Imperial Russia. Such rapid advances have been decidedly uneven, in terms of basic human needs. However, every developing country has its own unique and often intertwined factors which influence both its economic performance and progress in occupational health.

China is the fastest growing and most successful developing economy, with more than 112 million people directly involved in manufacturing. Much of Chinese industrial advance has been due to the so-called TVEs, or Town and Village Enterprises, which employ more than 146 million workers [1] and are groups which promote industrial development in a variety of industries, often in the absence of large capital investment [2]. These enterprises have grown rapidly, with unskilled and ill-educated labour virtually straight off the land. This has resulted in a crude industrial infrastructure with little or no Health and Safety awareness or controls. Observations made more than a decade ago still are relevant in terms of a lack of management awareness or interest in safety, lack of worker knowledge of these issues, uncontrolled and unmeasured hazardous processes and practices, as well as lack of safety in basic workplace facilities in terms of fire escapes, ventilation and other essentials [3]. Several industries, such as mining, shoe manufacture, metal finishing, as well as plastics manufacture have high incidences of worker injuries, as well as causing untold problems in the future due to the toxicity of metals, solvents and combinations of toxic materials [3]. Indeed, in China it is not unusual to see images and accounts of modern and large factories producing a range of goods from paper to pharmaceuticals, discharging effluent into a river which is actually the only source of drinking water for the local inhabitants [4]. If billions are invested into high-technological manufacturing process development, whilst perhaps a mile or so down the road people are wading out of a river with a few filled buckets to drink and wash, it is hardly surprising that Occupational Health and Welfare has not yet evolved to the level where it can protect workers effectively.

India possesses a comparable population to that of China, but in contrast, only 26 million people work in 'organised' occupations such as those seen in the developed world. Just over 11 million are directly involved in manufacturing [5], although even for this relatively modest number, there is only half the Medical and Safety Officer complement required by India's long-standing occupational health legislation to serve these workers' needs. The rest of India's working population is involved in what is termed the 'informal' economy, which ranges from agricultural labour, either paid or at a subsistence level, to countless other manual labouring occupations [6]. The combination of very low healthcare and occupational health expenditure, poor or non-existent enforcement of occupational legislation, a general lack of regulation and the sheer physical danger and toxicity associated with many of these occupations contribute to the estimated 403 000 work-related deaths per annum in India [7].

Among the growing Latin American economies, Brazil, with its wealth of natural resources, embraced manufacturing much earlier than most developing countries, although its share of the economy has actually fallen since the 1980s and 1990s to a current involvement of around nine million people. Consequently, worker's rights and health provision are far more advanced in Brazil than most developing countries, as around 33% of workers are protected by the National Institute of Social Insurance, which provides compensation for work-related injuries and disabilities. This system is backed by inspections of working premises and paid for through a levy on private companies known as *Seguro Acidentes de Trabalho* (SAT), or Work Injuries Insurance [8]. However, even with such a system, younger workers are not as well protected as other groups, and they are subject to high rates of injury [8]. Whilst strenuous efforts are being made around the world to encourage occupational health infrastructure development [9], as well as practical and successful local initiatives to improve worker safety [10], it is sobering to consider that whilst 148 fatal work-related accidents were reported in the UK between 2012 and 2013 [11], more than 47,000 such deaths were estimated to have occurred in India in 2003 alone [7]. Overall, it has been estimated that the total number of work-related premature deaths in developing countries annually exceeds 1.8 million [7].

It is to be hoped that political, economic and even moral pressures will cause the evolution of better legal structures which will allow more workers in the developing world to gain some redress for their injuries. Countries such as China, Brazil and India already have large and prospering Higher Education, as well as Research and Development sectors, and these will be part of the creation of a future infrastructure for training in hazardous substance handling and Occupational Medicine, as well as Health and Safety. These factors will eventually bring these and other emerging economies to the top table of world exporters, who manufacture sustainably and profitably, whilst safeguarding the health of their workforces.

References

1. Chinese Ministry of Agriculture. 2001–2007 Report of Development Agriculture in China [in Chinese]. Beijing, China: Chinese Ministry of Agriculture, 2008.
2. Wang PX et al. Occupational health and safety challenges in China–focusing on Township-Village enterprises. Arch Environ Occup Health, 66(1), 3–11, 2011.
3. Brown GD. China's factory floors: an industrial hygienist's view. Int J Occup Environ Health. 9, 326–339, 2003.
4. Kaiman J. Inside China's 'cancer villages' June 4th, 2013. http://www.guardian.co.uk/world/2013/jun/04/china-villages-cancer-deaths (accessed on 18 November 2013).
5. Sharma K et al. Need and supply gap in occupational health manpower in India. Toxicol Indust Health. 29, 483–489, 2013.
6. Pingle S. Occupational safety and health in India: now and the future. Ind Health. 50, 167–171, 2012.
7. Al Tuwaijri S et al. XVIII World Congress on Safety and Health at Work, June 2008, Seoul, Korea – Introductory report – beyond death and injuries: The ILO's role in promoting safe and healthy jobs; International Labour Office. – Geneva: ILO, 2008.
8. Santana VS et al. Workdays lost due to occupational injuries among young workers in Brazil. Am J Ind Med. 55, 917–925, 2012.
9. Peres F, Claudio L. Fifteen years of occupational and environmental health projects support in Brazil, Chile, and Mexico: a report from Mount Sinai school of medicine ITREOH program, 1995–2010. Am J Ind Med. 56, 29–37, 2013.

10. Adams JSK et al. Increasing compliance with protective eyewear to reduce ocular injuries in stone-quarry workers in Tamil Nadu, India: a pragmatic, cluster randomised trial of a single education session versus an enhanced education package delivered over six months. Injury-Int J Care Injured. 44, 118–125, 2013.
11. Statistics on fatal injuries in the workplace 2012/13. Full-year details and technical notes. Health and Safety Executive. http://www.hse.gov.uk/statistics/pdf/fatalinjuries.pdf (accessed on 11 November 2013).

'Never get out of the boat, absolutely goddamn right. Unless you were going all the way.'

Captain Benjamin L. Willard,
in 'Apocalypse Now'
Directed and Produced by Francis Ford Coppola, United Artists, 1979.

Index

Expert Report Writing in Toxicology: Forensic, Scientific and Legal Aspects,
First Edition. Michael D. Coleman.
© 2014 John Wiley & Sons, Ltd. Published 2014 by John Wiley & Sons, Ltd.